I0099954

PLURAL SEX

CASE STUDIES IN VARIANT SEXUAL PRACTICES

by

CARSON DAVIS

The Borgo Press
An Imprint of Wildside Press LLC

MMIX

Copyright © 1969, 2005, 2009 by Carson Davis

All rights reserved.
No part of this book may be reproduced in any form
without the expressed written consent
of the author and publisher.
Printed in the United States of America

www.wildsidepress.com

SECOND EDITION

CONTENTS

INTRODUCTION

In our modern day and age, with sexual mores changing, with a total open freedom of attitudes, actions and expressions becoming the standard, it is not surprising to discover that almost any kind of sexual or "family" relationship is up for grabs. People are trying to express themselves in a manner that gives them the greatest amount of happiness and fulfillment.

Young men and women, today, find themselves living in a strange and frightening world, one that is becoming smaller and more compact and far less desirable than the one their grandparents grew up in. Today the international terrorists are creating a mood of fear that touches everybody in the civilized world. There is a frenetic search for experience and self-expression that is completely personal. There is a hungry cry to survive, live, find some kind of Utopia before life is stripped from the world in which we live. The young don't need the little wars to make the outlook for their future seem unpromising. They don't need the evidence that the fantastic birth rate might, in their time, may over-populate the world—if mankind *does happen* to survive! They don't need to look further than the front pages of their local newspaper, cable television or the Internet to realize how disorganized the future of the world promises to be. They need look no further than the immediate surroundings of their hometown to know that life is not a forever thing, and marriage is slowly becoming a mockery where promises are not kept.

Legal and illegal immigration has become the wave of not tomorrow but of everyday life. Human migrations are flowing across national borders as if they don't even exist. This, alone, is changing the very structure of life on this world. The old way is slowly fading to be replaced by a totally different kind of international society. In actual fact it is almost impossible to avoid. This is the natural evolution of humanity stretching itself across the face of a world of limited resources. Change is the norm; it is a shifting of power from haves to have-nots. It has always been so, but not on such a grand scale.

What does a young person think when they hear about the lack of job opportunities of their less fortunate friends?

What does a young person think when they hear about summer riots, discontentment in our own government toward international policies that might take them across the world to die in some rice paddy or desert wasteland for people they know little about and care less about than they do for the social unrest of our own country?

The young of today can look at the divorce rates and wonder if marriage is the final solution. They can see articles, books, read in the newspapers, hear on television and talk radio, about the changing moral attitudes of not only the United States, but the world in general.

Many rigidly fanatical religious conservatives will always scream unbendingly about moral ethics, about right to life, while the rest of us battle over just how liberal we should go concerning abortion, sexual conduct and lifestyles. Aids curved some major social habits, and dramatically changed a lot of ideas regarding relationships, while the gay community has pressed for legalized marriage between same sex couples. All of this came into our lives like a hammer smashing down to crush ideas and values and attitudes concerning how we should react to one another. The concept of tolerance to different ideas other than our own has become a rigid block to a more loving society in the twenty-first century.

Many things have changed since this book was originally published; but not everything. Back then, and now, many people were shocked to learn how suburban married couples form sex clubs where husbands and wives change partners for the night. The idea of swinging and poly-marriages are not new, just more openly debated.

With the facts, in simple order, bearing out a new truth about life and the society in which they live, it's no wonder that new moral and sexual attitudes are becoming widely practiced. This has not changed much in the past decades.

For the people interviewed in this book the "cold war" still existed, where atomic war could have wiped modern civilization off the face of the world. Today we have terrorism threatening our very existence, through the suicide bombings. A single fanatic might decide to blow themselves up in a populated area, killing as many people as possible. These were and are very serious realities that must be faced on a daily basis.

So even with the real threat of AIDS, which can be a death sentence, people are seeking new ways to relate. Too many people live with idea of enjoying their lives to the fullest before it is all over. And one finds it difficult to blame them. It isn't a matter of what is moral or right, in their minds, so much as resolving the question: what difference does it matter, if life is so short?

Pre-marital, extra-marital and swapping partners were never really new; throughout history they have happened to one degree or another. Each culture developed its own sexual attitudes, its own psychological hang-ups.

The Roman Empire is a prime example of a society that had totally different standards from our own.

Historically young girls willingly do their "patriotic

duty" in giving the boys in the armed forces one last fling before going into battle. War has always brought a more open attitude toward sexual adventures. Tomorrow we may all be dead, is the logic.

Today, with war unpopular, yet exploding in all the headlines, the young are examining their culture. They are facing up to the reality of the complex civilization in which they live, and are finding a new front, a new answer, one that the people in this book feel will become as common as the union of two people in holy marriage.

Examining other viewpoints always opens us to be less prejudice against people with different belief-systems from our own. In a world such as today it is a much-desired attitude that must be ultimately accepted; otherwise universal conflict will be self-destructive to all.

In simple terms: Plural sex means the sharing of living quarters, food, sex and any other item which makes up the living-unit with at least one other couple.

In today's society the expense of owning a home can be out of the reach of many couples, and they double and triple up in order to buy a house they equally share. What else goes on behind locked doors may not be much different from what is revealed in these case histories.

One man told me this: "Take your wife-swapping couples; they are being dishonest and unrealistic. They have to support different households. They are doing exactly what we do, but in a dishonest, unrealistic way. We don't fool ourselves: we say in effect: If we're going to swap mates, then let's get together, live together, share expenses and make the most of things as they are—not as we might think society demands it to be. Because of this, we can live a lot cheaper, get more for our money, and we don't have any sexual hang-ups."

While the part about sexual hang-ups is true as far as he was concerned, it was not true in every case. Each person had their own story to tell, and because of this I have organized the book in sections, complete in themselves, where each person reveals their own attitudes about life, sex and the other people they are living with. In order to get a total picture, I had each person go into some detail about his or her early sex life and reveal how they had finally decided that plural sex was their answer to personal happiness.

It is enough to say that I met one of the members of this sexual combine in the normal course of social contacts, and because all those she was living with were rebels it wasn't difficult to convince them to tell their story.

What makes this more interesting is the fact they are average people, holding down average jobs, going about their business of living much the same, on the surface, as any other group of people. The difference is simply they lived together and shared with one another in every way, emotionally, spiritually, intellectually, and sexually. They appeared to be one big happy, communal family.

—Carson Davis
2007

PLURAL SEX, BY CARSON DAVIS

CHAPTER ONE

LAURA

Laura is in her middle twenties, has attended college, but not completed it. It would take a second look to notice that she is actually a fairly nice-looking, well-shaped young woman, because she gives the appearance of being shy, plain, and unconcerned about her dress; in actual fact she stands about five-feet-five-inches, has dark brown hair, dark blue eyes, a rather straight nose, but pouty lips. Her body is trim of all fat, but thrusting in the bust line and her hips are well-formed curves that blend down nicely into lovely thighs and legs.

I saw her once in a two-piece bathing suit and was surprised how sensual she could appear, if she made any attempt to present her body in a fashionable manner. She usually dresses in loose-fitting blouses and flaring skirts that reveal little of her sexual attractiveness. She speaks with a slight English accent, which comes from the fact that she was born in England, but has lived in the United States since she was ten years old. Her "A" is "ah", but there is little about her that is actually affected, in fact she's quite the opposite. I learned that in college she took up dramatics with the hope of being an actress, quickly given up after about six months study.

I met her some years ago, when she was just "off" the

acting bit, though she had the theatrical habit of throwing her arms about you and affectionately kissing your lips, then saying "darling" after every statement directed toward a man. We lost track of one another and only a few months ago met again, at which time I learned about her immediate social life—one which proved interesting enough to question her in detail. Because of this meeting and the ones that followed, it became possible to put together the following case histories.

After having interviewed her mutual roommates, I edited the material into a series of dialogues which gave each person's evolution toward the communal living they mutually share. [The rest are offered in this series of *The Carson Davis Files.*] Hers was the first, since she was one of the "founders" so-to-speak of their living arrangement with other couples in the same, shared house. She was there at the very beginning.

Now, to let Laura tell her own story:

* * * * * * *

I guess it wouldn't shock you to learn that sex has been an important thing to me since I was a teenager. When you met me I was carrying on a passionate affair with your friend, a fact hardly secret, since we were living together at the time. But, be that as it may, it was only one of many such affairs which led me to the present conclusions about life and how I want to live.

If I've learned anything about living, it's simply that if you don't grab a large chunk of life for yourself, nobody is going to give it to you.

This world in which we live is such a damned lie. It really made me mad to discover what a lie everybody is living. You know how it is. People say one thing and they mean the other.

For as long as I can remember, Mom was telling me

how demanding men were. I mean that she was always implying that sex was a four-letter word that wasn't any fun and she just wouldn't think of enjoying it, no matter what! I didn't realize at the time she was a terrible speller! Sex a four-letter word? How dumb could she be?

But it wasn't long before I learned what a lie *that* was. I'll never understand how our mothers could tell such lies about themselves and about life. You'd think it would be their duty to give the real facts of life to their children, rather than painting a picture that wasn't true.

I guess every child remembers some time or other when they've been told, either in words or by implication, that sex is dirty. You know how it is. They say you shouldn't touch yourself "down there." And you shouldn't "do that" until you get married. They won't come out and even use such gentle words as sex organ or sexual intercourse. Of course, I don't know how I might have reacted if one of my parents had used the word sex in that way. But if they'd been different right from the start, I might not have found it embarrassing.

If I found a kid of mine masturbating, well, I'd try to make him or her think it was the most natural thing in the world; not make a big thing out of it. Know what I mean?

It doesn't take a girl long to learn the facts of life, if that's what she wants. What takes so long is understanding there are facts worth learning about. You, you hear about the birds and the bees—oh, boy, that's a lovely one. Every man is just a little bee, flitting from bird to bird—doesn't make sense at all. Oh, sting, sting, that hurts, love!

I just get sick and tired of hearing cute little words for the real thing.

The other day I was talking to an old girl friend of mine. We hadn't seen each other for ages—we'd been in high school together and then drifted apart, after I'd learned what it felt like to have a big fat dick in my snatch. This girl hadn't ever had sex! Can you imagine, over twenty-one and not having had your cherry bombed out? She said: "I just couldn't let a boy do that to me." I laughed and asked what she meant by "that." Her face blushed and she said: "You know, doing what married couples do!"

So I just bombed her out and asked: "You mean, dicking your snatch?"

She didn't understand what I meant. So I said it this way: "Screwing your pussy?"

The whole girl seemed to blush. I couldn't believe it. I guess I was being a little nasty—and to be quite honest, putting it on pretty thick. We talked for some time after that and I finally told her she was really missing something.

What bombed me out was the fact she'd never even *seen* a man's dick.

I remember when I first saw a man's penis, and it was quite a surprise, I'll tell you, because I shouldn't have even been there. It was a horrible shock at the time.

I came home early from school, because I wasn't feeling too well. I didn't make much noise and as I was going down the hall to my room, thinking there wasn't anyone else home, I heard these strange sounds in my folks' bedroom. A little concerned and frightened, I might add, I tiptoed down the hall to the entrance of the folks bedroom. The door was half open and the sight that met my eyes really bombed me out, but good.

Remember what I said about my dear old mommy saying that sex wasn't so nice...well, for a woman who didn't like it, she was showing great signs of being a very good actress, without any lessons or experience in acting.

Here my lovely, and she is lovely, even now, for her age, mother was naked as we all are born, flat on her back, legs spread wide and this guy doing push-ups right between them.

I stood there, both fascinated and horrified. I pretty

much knew what was going on, but couldn't keep my eyes away from what was happening. It would have been shocking enough to see Mom and Dad doing such a thing. But this bastard was *a total stranger,* somebody I'd never seen before and I learned that Mom hadn't seen before that afternoon.

Suddenly the two of them, making wild animal grunting sounds, slapped together, straining for all they were worth, then the man suddenly lifted up and I saw his big manhood sticking up like a sausage between his legs. Mom, still not seeing me there, whipped up and started going ape on his dick, as if her lips couldn't get enough of it.

At that point I just gagged, too shocked to believe what was happening.

Like I said, I was really bombed out, in every way. I gave out a little sick cry and turned, running out of the house as fast as I could go. I don't know much of what happened after that, other than I continued to run until exhausted, then walked, dazed beyond any rational thought. I just kept thinking what a fink Mother was, how she had lied to me, how she was cheating on Dad—everything that can go on in a girl's mind after seeing such a scene.

Every concept of so-called morality was finished from that day on. I walked until it was dark and then continued to walk. I don't know if I ever really planned on picking some guy up or not. I guess I never even thought of anything but the horror of that bedroom scene with Mother screwing a strange man. I hated her.

You see, a girl grows up being virgin in mind and body, then suddenly all the stories you've heard are proven false, a lie!

I was fifteen, and fairly matured for my age, even then. Physically, that is. I'd dated boys, but never done more than neck and to me that meant just that: nothing lower than the neck.

I was walking down the main drag of town when a

couple of boys I knew at school came out of a drug store. They called to me, asked what was wrong. I guess my face was still tortured by what I'd seen.

One of them had been hot for my tail for months, and he had a reputation of being a real lover-boy, so I'd cooled it with him. But this night, when he started talking to me, I began to think that maybe there was something to sex, maybe I should just go get me a good piece of male. Of course, I didn't think of it in that way, then, but it amounted to just that.

He finally got to asking me if I wanted a ride home.

I looked directly into his eyes and said: "Not home, but I'll take a ride with the two of you, any place you want to go."

I must have purred out the last in a very sexy way. It got my message across.

Derk—that's the lover-boy's name—he winked to his buddy and then grinned real hard at me.

"Anywhere?" he asked, taking my arm, squeezing it like he already knew the answer.

Without batting an eye I simply said: "Anywhere and we can do anything you want. I feel very cooperative. That's what you've been wanting, isn't it?"

A girl can't be much more obvious. I might as well have said, let's go fuck like mad!

He said something to the effect, "Crazy, real crazy!"

We went to his car and I sat in the back with his buddy, who wasn't the shy type. He was all hands, first on my arm, shoulder, then he ran a finger down to my thigh. I just sat there numb, not caring—yet, caring *very* much! When he lifted up my skirt and played his fingers up between my legs, at the same time cupping one of my breasts and kissing my lips, the fires of real passion spurted.

I didn't give a damn what they thought of me. It didn't matter any longer.

When he got his fingers up to the elastic of my panties,

I helped, lifting my fanny so he could work them off my body. He worked real fast and before I knew it he was fingering my snatch and that felt damned good.

Remembering what a man looked like, I just reached out and felt between his legs to discover he had a real fat hard pressing against his pants. *That* was exciting! My, but he was so hard. I hadn't imagined that a man could feel that hard. I wondered if it would hurt much.

He would have screwed me in the back seat right then, but Derk drew the car to a stop, turned, laughed, said: "Save it for the house, friend!"

We were parked outside Derk's home. His parents were away for the week, on vacation. It was a great set-up.

Of course this wasn't the time for thinking about such things. All I could think of was seeing my mother with that man. I have often wondered what made me do what I did with the two boys. Johnny, a boy friend of mine who was studying psychology, claimed I was trying to get even with Mom. But I don't think it was just that. I'd been burning with sexual desires that had been held in, because it was supposed to be the right thing to do. I would keep thinking, what would Mommy think? Now I knew it didn't *matter* what she thought. Fuck her!

We went into Derk's home and they suggested we all get undressed. I didn't really know what to expect, but we all undressed and I was fascinated at seeing the boy's small weapons; like they weren't there. That is, at first. By the time they got a good look at my young breasts and snatch, their pricks started growing and *that* was fascinating!

We went into the master bedroom, where his folks had a large double bed. Laying down on it, the boys started caressing me and kissing my body. It was thrilling, like I'd never been thrilled before. They were touching me all over the place and when their hands started playing between my legs, I got so hot that I was panting with desire.

Derk laughed after a while and said: "She's ready, real ready!"

Then he climbed on top of me and started rubbing his big fat hard against my snatch. I just rubbed up against the big stick between his legs, just like I'd seen Morn doing, and I knew then why she'd been so crazy.

Kids know nothing about sex. But they learn fast. When Derk stuck himself into me, it hurt, I'll tell you that, but it felt terrific, too. He was pretty good for a kid, and made the most of it. I almost climaxed by the time he filled me. Then the other guy got his turn and I really came. Derk was sucking my tits while his pal was dicking me deep and fast and I was just crazy and started clawing around between his legs. When his pal was finished, Derk was ready to pop and I half dragged him to me. We united real fast and I just rode faster and faster on his stick until the lights went out.

The two boys thought I was great. Derk said he'd been surprised to learn I was a virgin. I laughed and stated that wasn't so any more.

That night when I got home, real late, Dad was furious. He sent me to my room and was going to paddle me good, but I turned on Mom and just blurted out that I'd simply done what she'd been doing with that strange man in the bedroom.

Dad's fury turned on Mom. I had never seen him really mad before, but now he leaped at her like some insane animal, striking her face back and forth. I was so frightened that I called the cops. By the time they got there, Dad and Mom were simmered down, sitting, staring at each other like dumb beasts. I never knew why they didn't get a divorce. I guess they made some kind of arrangement. But things were never the same after that. I wouldn't have anything to do with Mom and became very close to Dad.

Funny, I've never thought much about it before, but I

didn't have too many sexual experiences after that. You'd think it would naturally follow. But...I would date boys and when they'd start getting fresh with their paws, I'd cool it. Though there were a few guys I let stick my snatch in high school.

I remember one, a real big guy, and he looked large as hell between his legs. We dated a couple of times, and I was so turned on by him, so interested in learning how big he really got, that I couldn't control myself when we started necking one night in the car.

My hand just ran down between his legs and felt the largest hard I've ever felt in my life. Hell, he was over six feet tall, all muscle, real broad shouldered and his prick was like a mile long and steel all the way. I was fascinated. It twitched in my fingers and suddenly he ran his own hand up my skirt and found the place where my panties pulled tight over my snatch. He tried to wiggle a finger under the panties and the pleasure that brought was just too much.

I started helping him and suddenly he was really caressing my pussy, pumping his finger in deep to explore. Finally I couldn't stand that much longer, so I unzipped his fly, got his large fat tool out and worked it up and down with my hand. We were really going to town on each other—but masturbation wasn't what I wanted—I just had to discover what it felt like having such a big prick in me. The whole idea seemed delicious. It's funny, though: I've learned you don't have to have a large one to give a girl a great big thrill. It's what you do with it that counts. But this guy knew what to do, too.

He lifted me up, straddled my legs over him, then lowered me down until the tip of his large shaft was just touching my snatch. I trembled to get it in me, but his big strong arms held me so that all I could feel was the large crown, and that drove me wild. Laughing, he finally slowly lowered me until I was having a climax just from the lovely size and length of his tool. But it was a little climax—I guess more in my mind than anything else.

Geeze, when I think about that. It was a real groovy screw. Once he was in me we just sorta jerked against one another and it was great. After it was over I did what Mom had done, and I understood what had driven her to it. I lowered my head and started kissing and kissing that wondering tool of his like I couldn't get enough.

We dated a few more times, and I remember when we were out in the country, screwing on a blanket…he had positioned himself on top and he teased me with that big weapon, just using the crown on my snatch, then when I just went out of my mind, completely bombed out, he thrust deep, almost choking me with the raw sensation.

I thought he would ram up right through my body. But I took all he had to give and felt I could have taken more.

Outside of him, there was another guy, but he didn't matter, just a one-night stand.

I was hot and bothered, tired of playing with my snatch for weeks on end. I wanted a dick. So when this boy next door—he was visiting his aunt and uncle—came over and just wanted to be friendly, I managed to make it more than friendly. I don't know what got into me. But we were talking on the front lawn and suddenly I said: "Let's go someplace where we can be alone."

He wasn't so good looking, but I didn't care. We went to the park, talked and when it was fairly dark we ended up in the bushes, screwing the hell out of one another.

But I was seventeen by then and high school was almost finished off—so that was the last of the sex parties I experienced before hitting college.

I knew about sex, and I knew what a great pleasure it could be, but living at home, with too many people knowing the family, I just didn't want to go all ape. Even with the folks knowing about me—and they didn't dare try to stop my activities.

Dad had had a talk with me after that first time, he'd told me a few of the real facts of life.

I mean that he told me how babies were born and things like that—which I knew pretty much about—but then he told me that there were ways to protect yourself. That was very important because after that I knew it was possible to have all the men I wanted, without getting babies.

Yet, as I said, I didn't really start making the rounds until I hit college.

Oh, boy, brother. I'll tell you there is quite a difference between high school sex and what goes on in college! A girl just can't imagine how different it is. You think because you've had it a few times, you know the score. But I had a lot to learn.

It really bombed me out, in every way.

I didn't know anything about some of the "different" things that can go on. I thought a guy popped one in and then that was it. Or you could have something like a romance that would be love. Strangely, I'd never really thought much about that in high school. Boys were something to take you out to movies and dances and things like that—not to love. I didn't even really get a crush on any guy. Guess that's because I'd learned what it was about— or thought I did—and getting all shot up because I had hot pants for a boy and didn't know what to do with myself. Shit! Remember how some of the girls—the prudes, afraid of sex—would get all hot and bothered and think they were in love.

Boy, I can tell you about love.

I know some people would think that a girl who lives like I do...well, the squares think that you could hardly jump in bed with one guy, while loving it with another. You were a slut, whore. Cheap lay. Well, there's all kinds of love, and I've learned something about *that,* too. Gosh, you can love a man's hard, nothing more and just go ape

21

over it. You can fondle and kiss and tug it between your lips like you can't get enough of what it can give you. You can just *love* that!

You can love a guy because he thinks great. Real, real great like Dave...he started out being a little too intellectual about sex, I put him wise to that.

That's one of the things about living with another couple or more, like we do. The gals and guys learn how to interrelate, not on a one to one basis, but on a community basis. You learn the difference and the different needs each person has. Sometimes I want to be with Dave like I can't stand it. Not to sex it up, mind you, though that happens a lot because we have a thing about getting together. I admire and just love his brain, while he's learned to like the kind of sex I'm willing to put out. He told me one night, while caressing my stomach—we'd loved it up real great a little bit before and we were naked as we'd been born, alone in the house, because the others were out working...we have the same day off...which is just great. But, anyway, he told me that because of having made the scene with me, he'd learned that sex can mean more than mere orgasm while at the same time *be* pure orgasm. That really bombed me out, because I didn't dig what he meant.

He said: "Honey, before I knew you, I thought it was all romance, love and kisses—even when I joined our group I still had this idea that a guy had to be totally involved with a girl...because *she* had ideas of romantic involvement. You know what I mean about that...while you're with a girl, it should mean something deep. But now I know it can be mere orgasm, nothing more. *But it still has to be with a girl you really care about.*"

See what I mean? He digs sexing me, because I'm wild. I don't pull any punches about wanting to come on strong with a man. But there is something great when you really feel strongly about him. Yet, at the same time, you're sexing for orgasm, mutual pleasure—but with a stronger kick.

We learn from one another. I learn more than the sex thing with David. He has a great mind.

But I've gotten off the bit. In college I had to grow, in many ways.

I hadn't fallen for a man. Nothing merely romantic. I wanted sex, so I finally gave in and let something happen. That was the high school kid. I wanted to go to a movie, so I got some guy to take me to one. But in college you have a totally different scene.

For one thing, you're in a new world. When you first take up quarters at the dorm, you don't know anybody and you're frightened silly. You're on your own and everybody else is in the same boat. So, you start desperately making friends. But the friends are strangers. Well, they haven't grown up with you. You hardly know the girls and you suddenly find that you know them better than you'd known some from back home.

Well, that sounds confusing, I know, but what I'm saying is that the girls get down to the nuts and balls of it all.

You start finding girls who think the same way you do. I remember having a conversation with a group of girls, maybe it was my third or fourth day in college, and they started talking about sex, and it became apparent that all of us had had men one time or another. My own experiences were just about average. Some girls only had it once, some dozens of times.

Well, one of the girls, who had been to the college the year before, knew the places to go, what guys to meet and how to make the whole scene.

She offered to take us to a place where we'd meet the swinging crowd.

That night, after going to this beer joint, where they blasted the juke box and couples danced, I ended up with some guy who had a real good line and a real great way of dancing. He'd look at me like he was undressing my body, sure of himself. He knew this was exactly what would happen, too. And he was right.

To be truthful, by that time, I was hot to really have a real man. It had been some months—well, maybe over a year—since I'd had a good lay. I didn't know any better way to make friends...like, if you don't run with the right group, you don't get things happening to you.

Oh, I've heard the arguments that a girl doesn't have to sleep with boys in order to become popular. And I've seen that rule proven. As well as disproved. Some girls won't sleep with guys and they are very popular; some will, and they have a hard time. There are some girls who are balling it all the time, but are very unhappy. I really don't see where it makes any difference. Every girl has to make up her own mind.

You know, I've heard guys complain that it isn't supposed to be manly to cry—well, maybe I should put it another way. They have been told that men don't cry, only that girls can cry, and they complain how a girl's got it made. Did they ever think how a girl is told time and time again, from the first moments of awareness of such things, that she isn't supposed to give herself to a man...that she's supposed to bottle all her physical and emotional needs and keep them corked up tight?

That's the trouble with the world today, too many dos and don'ts. If people were only taught to be realistic about themselves.

If we're hungry, we should eat. No matter what the hunger is. Well, outside of hurting somebody. Unless both you are with a person who wants the hurt scene. That's difference, I suppose. But if it's sex, pleasure, why not have a good helping of it, simply because it feels good and is good for the body and the emotions—and mind.

One girl told me: "I mentioned to Mom that sometimes I just could hardly control myself, wanting to touch a man down there. She told me, Honey, it's perfectly normal. and you're old enough to know the score about sex and what makes babies. If you really like a boy and want something to happen, just do what you want...if you desire touching him in an intimate manner, just go on ahead and do it. Ever since then, when I wanted to squeeze a man's prick, I did just that. Squeeze away!"

I thought this was just a great statement to make. Hell, if you want to reach down and start feeling a dick and balls, what's to stop you?

When this boy suggested we split the place, I was more than ready. I was hot all over.

He had a real pad, not far from the place we'd been drinking and dancing and we went to it. It was a pad, I meant that. He was an arty type guy—and he had a way of living that had style: huge modern pictures on the wall, low sofa, and a scattering of large colorful pillows on the floor. There was a small bar in the corner and a hi-fi set behind it. He put on the music, one with a beat, and fixed us highballs, then indicated the low couch where we sat close together. Almost immediately he started talking sex. I remember quite a bit about this night, because he was my first college dick.

I remember his first important question—important to me, because it made sexual intercourse easy to fall into:

"You dig sex, Laurie?" He had his arm about my shoulder and I felt his fingers squeeze my arm.

"It's part of life, isn't it?" I offered, feeling high and excited. I could see right then, between his legs, was a big beautiful hard just waiting to give me a lot of pleasure. How I wanted to feel that with my fingers. I remembered what this girl had told me...the advice her mother had given—and I decided I'd just reach down and explore. But at the right moment.

Funny, most guys don't understand that a woman is much like a man, really. She has a brain and a body that responds to sexual ideas. Sure, she doesn't fire up as fast as men—but under the right circumstances, she can be as hot to get on with the basic screwing as he is. I mean, a girl can actually be way ahead of him, maybe having experienced some juicy orgasms that revved her up real good …be so ready.

Well, my statement about sex being a part of life sparked him, almost immediately…but into conversation.

"Sex with the right girl is something wild. I mean that it all has to be just right and I think romantic to some degree, don't you?" Like that, he talked.

What could I say, but: "I guess there's nothing wrong with romance."

"Well, you meet a girl and you find her real exciting and beautiful and you really want to make it with her, but you don't know what she wants, so you have to play it easy. See what I mean? Like with some girls it would be easy to just bring them up here and say strip down honey, we're going to have a party. With other girls you just don't know what to expect."

If I'd known what he was leading up to, I might have been miffed in a different way. He sounded so damned slow. I wanted to be sexed, romanced, but sexed, most of all. He was overdoing the talk-part of my seduction. I learned later that this was a little game he played. Some girl, I can't remember who, told me he dug getting a chick hot and bothered to the point where she started making the advances.

I fell right into it.

There we were on the couch, two big drinks in our hands, my body hot and his damned prick stiff and large between his legs. If his zip had been yanked open and his donger exposed, it would be a big flag pole pointing like a thick arrow at the ceiling!

Finally, after his conversation had gone on like, well, just saying what should or could happen, for several minutes, I just reached down between his damned legs and covered that hard stick.

"Gee," I said, "that's really big. Where'd that come from? You're huge!"

"What do you think it should be? You're an exciting girl, I'm excited by you." He squeezed my shoulder again, and I wanted him to squeeze my whole body.

"I think," I suggested boldly, "that I'd like to feel more of what you have hiding there!" I giggled, realizing how blunt that was. I was bombed out with need, by then! Oh, you have no idea how I wanted him stripped naked. Well, at least his meaty cock & balls!

He chuckled and said, "Help yourself." The offer drove my fingers to unzip him. The surprise came when I discovered he didn't have any underpants on. There his stick was, large and red-hot, thrusting out of his fly. Oh, I'll tell you, it looked wonderful. I fondled and squeezed and jerked on it, just thrilled to death. He lay back, pleased by my actions.

Suddenly I just couldn't take waiting around like that and I wanted more exciting thrills.

So I turned, coming into his arms. Without expecting to do so, I threw one leg over him and pressed my fully clothed snatch against his shaft. Oh, that felt just great. Too great, because I wanted to burst free of my clothing.

There's nothing like having a large, thick hard between your legs, or pressed up against your snatch. I just wanted to be naked against the lovely thick shaft of his. What a prick.

Just thinking about it makes me hot. I was flushed all over, and you can believe that my snatch was flushed full and hot with passion. You have to remember this was my first time with a man since that last quickie in high school. And, for me, this was the first time with a *real* man. I was on my own, free, and felt very mature and adult. Everything made me hot.

We kissed terribly passionately and his hands were all

over my body at once, breasts and fanny. Then I felt his fingers working my skirt up and I really went to town rubbing against his shaft, encouraging him to continue getting my skirt out of the way.

"Hurry, oh, please, hurry!" I moaned, starting to unbutton his shirt.

Gosh, I remember the excitement and thrills as his hands fondled my fanny, then pulled on my underpants, squeezing my naked butt. Suddenly I lifted up, standing on the sofa, in front of him. He got my skirt off and then pulled my panties down. I felt flushing excitement as he really gave my snatch a going over with his eyes.

I started doing things with my hips. You know, rolling them, then jerking, like a man was inside me and I was screwing him real good.

Suddenly he grabbed my hips and was burying his face against my hot moist snatch. Oh, his singing tongue just laced itself along all the nerves at once. I climaxed right there, shoving up against his face. Then suddenly lie urged me downwards. While doing this, he lowered full length on the sofa, lying on his back. I found my place just above his hard throbbing prick. Then blowsville. He was in, deep.

Funny that I should remember so much detail about that first time. But it almost feels like it's happening right now. That's something about sex, sometimes you don't remember one act from another—it fades—and the only thing that counts is the last one or, better yet, what's happening right at the moment.

Yet, I remember almost every sensation of what took place.

He was real large and when he penetrated me, I just screamed out in joy. It felt so good, tucked deep into my snatch like that. Then suddenly I had control. I'd never had control like this before. I just kept lifting up and dropping down, up and down, then circled my hips, just greedily working myself on that wonderful shaft of manhood.

He kept fondling and squeezing my breasts and it felt real good.

During the last moments, I simply went out of my bombed-out mind, clawing at him. I'd never felt so animal before in my life.

Afterwards we lay side by side, exhausted, until he started caressing my stomach and breasts and my nipples just became taut as hell, and he started moving his fingers along my stomach, while sucking my tits deep into his mouth, even hurting and biting a little with his teeth. That felt great. I really thrust up, wiggling hard against his hand when he covered my pussy, which was bursting with heat, by then.

All at once he was on top of me, brutally hammering his stick of love deep. I went ape, wrapping my legs around his, thrusting with his thrusts until one climax after another convulsed my own body.

I'll tell you one thing, there never was a happier girl than the one that left his pad that night.

We developed a thing for some time, then finally I met a boyfriend of his and at this party he was giving, this guy, Johnny by name, got me in the bedroom and we had a wild winging session. He had me on the bed and his hands were up my skirt, clutching to the naked flesh of my thigh, above the nylons. When he got himself naked from the waist down, and was pulling my panties off, I started going crazy. There had been a lot of drinks and the feel of his hot dick just bombed me out and I started eating away on him like he was some all-day sucker. When he'd gone off, he grabbed me, sat on the bed, threw me over his lap and started spanking my fanny, saying I was a very bad girl to have ruined a good thing. But the spanking was like nothing I'd ever experienced. It was erotic and his fingers started finding their place where they shouldn't have been. I'd never known I was erotically sensitive in the rear, but he probed until I was having a wild orgasm. I felt his stick up like a hot rod against me, and we suddenly tumbled on the bed and we frantically attempted to join our bodies. When it happened I climaxed almost immediately, because of all the things he'd been doing before.

My lover-boy, in whose pad we were balling it, stepped into the room, saw what was happening! He stood there watching, and when Johnny was finished, he replaced him. I was a little surprised at what happened, but climaxed almost immediately. They took turns with me and I took everything they had to offer.

Now I didn't want to be tied down to any one piece of action. From that moment on, for a couple of years, I was padding down with different guys.

All this might seem pretty wild to some folks. But you have to understand that when a girl is honestly learning about her body and her sexual needs, she will explore all types of lovers. Johnny had shown me that there were other ways to fly and I just had to learn *all* the ways to orgasm.

I guess I'd have to say the next years were explorations. They taught me a lot of things that became very important later.

Well, let me put it this way. You have so many ways to use a man's cock, and if a girl learns to be free-wheeling about sex, she has a better chance to live a fully satisfactory sex life.

I went to some real wild parties during this time. And when I think about my prudish ideas before getting to college, I shudder. I changed a lot during these two years. I believe for the better, because I'm far happier than most young women my age. I'm not afraid of sex, and I'm not afraid to talk to men about how I want it.

Let me explain that a little better.

Take this scene, as an example.

I was at a small banging party one evening with a trio

of other girls. We all sexed it up with boys, but the other girls were a little timid about what they wanted. One, June by name, was all for sex, but in privacy.

I laughed, lifted up my skirt and said, "First guy to get an erection can have this, right here!" Hell, I wouldn't have thought of doing such a thing years before. And, even though it sounds brutal, you have to understand I knew all the boys intimately and the girls had been screwed by them, in private. We were all pretty drunk and had been viewing some stag movies. One of the girls had been in the bedroom, screwing and I'd played between one of the boys' legs while the film was being viewed—but that was all in darkness.

So all of us had been talking about screwing in no uncertain terms. Maybe I should develop the scene this way:

After some conversation about sex, in general terms, one boy, call him Jack, said: "We're all mature, and we all know none here is a virgin. Why shouldn't we try something really wild?"

"Like what," one girl wanted to know, her face flushed with embarrassment.

"An orgy scene. Why not? There's no reason to be coy about it."

I asked: "Exactly what are you offering, gang-banging?"

Jack nodded and the other guys were all over it from the expression on their faces.

I looked at the girls and realized they needed a real kick in the ass, so to speak. I wanted to try this kind of thing out. Like I said, we were all pretty drunk. I figured the girls would put up, if somebody came out and really started the ball rolling. So I simply lifted up my skirt, challenging both boys and girls, saying, like I told you, "First guy to get an erection can screw me here and now."

If you consider what I was saying and my attitude, I can't say it is hard to understand why I said it that way. I didn't want to play any more games. I wanted sex, and I knew that having more than one guy at a time was just great. We were all mature and a little bit horny, by then. Like, you can't do something like that with kids, but with swinging adults you can do anything you want, and nobody is *really* going to be shocked. I didn't think of myself as sexually dirty, just realistic. Though, to be honest, I wouldn't do something like that now, I've learned there are better ways, like living in the same house with other couples and gang-banging as a natural course of life. You learn to have a mutual respect and...well, maybe it's even a form of deep affection for some of the people. You intercommunicate, you relate in a total way and aren't afraid to be yourself, no matter what that is, because everybody else is exactly the same as you: honest about their sexual needs.

Well, in any case, the other three girls took the tiger by the tail and started giving out with more blatant offers.

First a blonde said: "I'll go one better, boys." And she lifted her skirt, pulled down her panties and said: "See, I'm natural blonde. Don't you other girls want to reveal the true color of your hair?"

That knocked all of us out. Before three minutes had passed, all the girls were stripped and the boys beginning to follow our example.

Jack suggested we just take on the person to our right and see what happened.

It really happened that night, but it was nothing, really, against what happens many nights in our own little home.

But you have to understand it took me a long time to get to that point; I'd been to some wild parties before, and done the scene before that—in fact with the guy named Jack.

There are some real great college parties...ones where the music is full blast, the booze running free, and girls come without panties on, because they *know* what's going to happen!

You hang around, talking for some time, drinking and wondering if it is going to really swing. Then some guy either starts making passes or asks you to dance, and you start making with the sex plays.

I remember one guy who stepped up to me, looked at my body like he was making it naked, then reached out, lifted my skirt and grinned, saying: "Let's make it, pussy-cat."

I laughed, grabbed at his balls and we marched off into one of the bedrooms and screwed. I'd never met him before, but I was hot just looking at the guy. He'd been eyeing me for some time across the room and I'd grinned wantonly, hoping he'd make a play. That was a natural move—a little crude, lifting my skirt—but it made me turn on real fast, because there were a couple of other boys standing around, and they got a real great look at what this guy was going to possess. They really turned me on, and a little later each of them made a play that I accepted. I spent most of the time in the bedroom with one guy or another.

I know that sounds just terrible, if you think about it. But, really, if you know how I mean all this...well, some girls can have one man before they get married and they are whores—by their way of thinking—and somebody like me, well, can have a whole series of men and feel she is highly respectable.

Maybe the difference is that I'm never taken advantage of. You know, a girl who lets herself be seduced against her will, is nothing but a little tramp. I know that sounds backwards. But look at it this way:

She's kidding herself, claiming she doesn't want sex, while all the time she really does want it, so she either consciously or unconsciously lets men "seduce" her.

With somebody like me, well, I just admit I like sex, and when a man comes along who excites me, well, I swing.

No, that's not true. Not quite true, anyway. Not any-more. But it used to be, and I think it's healthy. If I hadn't learned about myself and what I felt about men and sex, I could never have arrived where I am today.

Isn't it enough to say that I've had a healthy sex life? Isn't it enough to admit that I've known men who like all kinds of sexual experiences. I know what different dicks feel like. I've done things like gang-banging and I've thrilled to having a man give me anal intercourse. I enjoy a little spanking now and then, because it's something dif-ferent.

But having had some detailed education about sex, I've gotten rid of my hang-ups and I'm not afraid of doing or trying anything. There are so many thrills to just letting yourself go.

I've known wives who are frightened to death to do anything really sexual—well, like playing with her man's prick, or putting it in her mouth. Some women are fright-ened if they let themselves go, be honest about sex, their husbands will be shocked.

One girl I know—married for about five years—is having an affair with another man. She told me it's the greatest thing that ever happened to her, because she just does all the things she wishes she could do to her husband.

Now, isn't that silly?

Why should a girl be afraid of being herself and just letting go?

You take our group. There are three couples and we started out simply by being social together. Jimmy, the guy I started living with. This other couple, Ann and Ralph, are married, but had been doing some swapping by the time they hit their second year of marriage. We got to socializing with them and then had a few real sex parties. Things were a little difficult for all of us, in the money de-partment, and we got to thinking how much fun it might be if we all lived together—renting a large house, to cut expenses.

So you see, it just worked out like that. Then we added a couple of other people and we've been having a real great life. Sometimes we have other couples staying at our house—like they join up, but after a while they split the scene.

But Jimmy, Ann, Ralphy, and me have been in it from the start and I'll tell you that Ralph is *really* a swinger.

He's a big boned guy, with large generous muscles that I just love to fondle and caress.

It's funny, now that I think of it, how things developed. You go dating, then start having an affair, then to face reality, you start living with a guy. Just like that.

Jimmy had a nice apartment, with a bedroom and owned his own furniture. So, I was having this affair with him—it was the first time I really dug a guy, for himself, though I haven't ever thought seriously of getting married to him, yet—and we were almost living at his place on weekends. He'd pick me up at work Friday, I'd fix dinner or we'd eat out, but end up in bed together, having an all-night orgy and then the next morning I'd cook breakfast and play house for the weekend. Finally it simply seemed logical that we start making it a full-time thing.

Well, here I was sleeping in my own apartment maybe twice a week. It was costing me hard bucks a month, so if we could save that, we'd have more money for other things. Have a bigger apartment, too!

When I lived at home, *before* learning about Mother, I would never have thought this would be possible. Up until then, I'd believed that home, family, husband was the natural future for a young woman.

But this seemed quite normal, natural. Neither of us really wanted to make it a forever thing, just desired being with one another. So we decided to simply shack up in his apartment.

Why not? It was the realistic thing to do.

I can't help but laugh about the first time I saw Ralph. He's a bull-necked guy, with a big body, a basic attitude about life. He likes to sit in front of the television set with a can of beer, watching sports. Jimmy isn't too much of a fan of sports, more slender and thoughtful, more interested in his electronics—which I don't really understand. But, anyway, we had Ralph and Ann over for dinner, and we all got sort of drunk and Ralph began getting real sexy with Ann. She's a big girl, has a more voluptuous figure than me...but her breasts sag a little—I guess you can't blame that on her. Funny thing about men, they want girls with big breasts, but want them to be firm and high on her chest. It's pretty hard to have both. He was sitting next Ann on the sofa, using his hand on her thigh. We got to talking about sex, and I guess that's pretty normal, when you come to think of it, most...young couples—in fact, older couples, come to of it—talk about sex most of the time, especially if they get drunk. Well, maybe not most of the time, but with our group, sex is an important part of life and we admit it. Instead of it bottled up inside, we just let it out.

Anyway, he said: "The trouble with most people is that they're afraid to admit they like...going to bed with one another—in public, I mean. Not doing it in public, you know, but...well...."

He gave Ann a savage look. "We've been married for a couple of years now and we really dig the bedroom...or living room, or even the shower."

He laughed at that and said: "You'd be surprised what a hot bed-partner Ann is."

Most girls would blush or be angry at her husband saying such a thing in public, especially when she hardly knew the other woman. It was the first time they had come over to our place. Jimmy had known Ralph for some time, but neither of them knew me.

She giggled and pressed her breasts against Ralph.

Jimmy glanced at me, grinned, and said: "Laura isn't one to be shy in such matters."

Ralph's eyes just burned me naked. *I* was the one to be embarrassed. I said there were a few things I had to do in the kitchen and went there to prepare the meal. I heard footsteps behind me some minutes later, and it was Ralph, who stood in the doorway staring at me in that raw sexy way of his.

He said: "You're really some dish."

I turned, found myself staring between his legs, startled at the realization he was hard up, and real large.

"Jimmy knows how to pick a woman," he announced. "Now, *you* I could go for."

"What about Ann?" I countered a little nervously, because suddenly I had the raw, naked desire to give his big hard a few squeezes.

"Oh, she wouldn't mind at all. We understand one another." He stepped close to me, placed a hand on the counter. I could have leaned forward and touched him.

"And what does that mean?" I countered.

Jimmy stepped into the kitchen then, said:

"They switch partners now and then."

Well, not being the kind to be easily shocked, I *was* a little surprised. Maybe a little pleased, too. In fact, I remember being very interested in Jimmy's statement and the way he searched my eyes. There was a questioning, a deep probing. I was certain he was wondering if I might go for such an arrangement.

I looked at Ralph, who was grinning down like the cat who is about to pounce on a mouse. I remember thinking: he would find a hot little trap if he tried to pounce on this little mouse; because I suddenly liked the idea of being caught by this ape of a man.

So I just said: "How interesting! Now that is something that sounds real interesting."

To make it short, let me put it this way. We talked

around it for no more than a few seconds and agreed it would be fun to have a real sex party; everybody was quite willing to go!

But it was a little different than one might expect.

I guess most people have heard of the game Sardines, but in case there are other ways to play it, I'll tell the ground rules we had: one person becomes the Sardine and they go find a place to hide—after the lights have all been turned out—then it is up to everybody else to find the Sardine. When normally played people get a little fresh with one another—accidentally, of course. Heaven forbid they'd touch a cock or tittie on purpose! Shocking thought! "Sorry about that!" "Oh, I just *know*, honey, darling, you didn't do it on *purpose*, any more than I meant my hand to be down there between your legs. My, my you're cock is *soooo* hard." Well, maybe not quite like that, but that's the unspoken gamesmanship of a different generation of Sardine players. The way we all play the game is thus: We all get naked and then the Sardine hides, once the lights are out then the others start looking for the Sardine. The game is supposed to be over when everybody has found the Sardine. Of course that makes for closed quarters, if somebody thinks of using a shower as a hiding place. And in the kind of game we play many times it ends up totally different from the conventional one, accidentally rubbed the dub, dub of your bum! Makes me laugh, really, people kidding themselves....

At the house with three or more couples it can be great fun. We'll have a full blasting party and invite other couples who have the more realistic ideas about sex and when we play Sardines, it can be *real* sexy. Groping and wiggling and squeezing and...you name it and it happens and no silly shit about being sorry about that. The only things we're sorry about is *not* having something to rub or touch or literally fuck!

With two couples, it isn't quite as exciting, but it's fun,

none the less.

Ann was the Sardine and we had to go find her, but before much time had passed, I felt groping hands reaching out and touching my fanny, then a finger probed between my legs, found a place against my crotch. Ralph's voice chuckled, then said: "*Thought* it wasn't Ann." Considering I'd been standing in the hallway, he could hardly have believed I was anybody other than Laura, of course. I giggled and reached down between his legs and fondled a real hard erection. "Guess you're not Jimmy, either!" I laughed, jerking on his hard prick all cocked up to fire. We stood there, hands on each other's privates, sexed up like hell. I was so bombed out I couldn't control myself. I simply pressed my hips against his prick, and our hands moved away. We were quickly kissing, tongues dancing back and forth and I captured his hard right between my thighs and started jerking back and forth.

Jimmy passed us, slapped my fanny, said:

"Let's find the Sardine!"

Ralph gently pushed me away and we made our search. Ann was lying on the double bed in our bedroom and when the three of us found her, it was sex-time. I managed to get Ralph and fairly drag him on top of me. We had a real goodie, I'll tell you. Afterwards we tried out a circus thing.

Well, if you think that's something. I remember when we had a party at the house with half a dozen couples and I was the Sardine and I went into the bathroom, getting in the tub. Finally a man found me and his hands made a real effort to identify my body in the darkness. I did the same thing to him, but couldn't tell who it was. But we managed to stretch out in the tub and begin screwing. Before we'd had an orgasm, some girl found us and then another girl and a man. But the sexing didn't stop and I didn't know who I was kissing or who kissed my breasts, whose prick I jerked off or went ape with, loving it up with lips and tongue or who was dicking me. It was a real orgasm and it didn't stop until everybody was in the bathroom, feeling and pawing, sexing and giggling. Oh, it was a real wild orgy.

In any case, I would like to say that Ralph, Ann and Jimmy served up some real sexy parties for quite a few months before we decided to join forces and live in a rented house together.

Once, I remember, climbing into bed, expecting Jimmy, and suddenly this big wonderful ape, Ralph was naked against me, his real hard between my legs, his hands pawing my breasts while his big tongue probed into my mouth. The unexpectedness of it was so exciting that I almost climaxed the minute his prick entered my hot pussy.

But I guess the real thing interesting is the way we all live.

Right now there are three couples. Dave, Nancy, Ralph and Ann, Jimmy and me. We girls take turns fixing meals, or do it together on weekends. The men take care of fixing household things and the garden. At night we usually watch television, either all together or in pairs or trios. There are three sets in the house—one is color. Each couple has a room to share, but we don't always share it with the same person.

Sometimes the girls will switch, going to one of the other men's rooms, or the men will surprise us by making an unexpected switch. Sometimes it is just a mutual thing—like you want sex with one of the other fellows.

Sometimes I want Dave, like I told you, and we have it on our day off together. But other times I need big ape Ralph. When one of us girls gets her period, the boys will sometimes gang up on the other two and it will be real fun. Then the girl with the period might just want some goodie. Once, knowing the boys were having a real session with Ann and Nancy, I couldn't keep my mind on the book I was reading. Ralph had dug anal intercourse, so I simply stripped down naked, went into the living room, where they were winging a real party and gripped the arms of a chair, wiggling my fanny in the direction of the boys, saying: "Who wants it this way! Come and get it!"

But usually when you have your period you don't go in for sex and generally when a girl is at that time of the month the others will be considerate and not have any real orgiastic party, but merely match up in private.

But what we have is a realistic arrangement where anybody can ask for goodies for the night with another partner, and you never get bored. Sex is something that is always different and interesting and if we want something even more different we'll invite some other couples over and have a real orgy. Sometimes even films to start things out.

I can't think of anything more to tell about our lives, other than the fact that when people are honest about their sexual urges they will face the fact that no *one* sexual partner is the living end. We have our fights and arguments among the couples and among each other, but there's always somebody there to turn to, to get understanding and affection from. And there is seldom any jealousy. If Jimmy gets mad at me, well he just goes to one of the other girls and I will sleep with whatever man is alone. We have a real wild time and it burns up the anger and hurt. Maybe the argument will last for a few days, so you sleep with this other guy until the fury burns out—or maybe you change back and forth between the two other men.

What can a married couple, living alone, do? The guy can go out and pick up some girl. Or she can do the same. But then you have a divorce staring at you—if things can't be worked out.

The nice thing about this is that you can walk out, go find a guy and get married if you want. But, as for me, I don't want. Not yet. Maybe I'll end up marrying Jimmy. I don't know. It doesn't matter, right now. I live, I'm happy, I can function as a total person, and I don't have the sexual hang-ups my parents had. Look at my mother. Boy, she almost blew the whole home apart. I still don't know how they managed to stick it out. But if they had been honest, maybe like I am, such a situation would never have happened.

I don't dig marriage built on lies and cheating. Where a married couple agrees that changing partners is healthy, then fine. That's living in the Now world; breathing freedom, living with your whole guts, as Ralph says.

To put it bluntly, as for me, there's no other way to live. Maybe in time I'll change, but I don't think so. I find this kind of life healthy, emotionally and physically.

As for having children; in time, maybe. But it will be planned and I'll know for sure who the father is. Like I said, sometimes I think it wouldn't be bad having a kid with Jimmy; but you have to get married. Ralph and Ann can't have kids, so they don't have anything to worry about. It's Ann, as far as I know—and Ralph couldn't care less about "brats" as he calls them.

Dave and Nancy are like us, living together, but not interested in making it a life-time thing, not at least in a legal sense. Dave told me, once, that marriage to him was unrealistic, binding, and that people had to be free agents—even if they love somebody very deeply.

Maybe that's right. At least for many people it *is* right! For me, I'm not worried. What happens in the future will be a natural outgrowth of what I am today. Everybody matures and changes, I guess, so I don't really know what my outlook will be tomorrow. I don't think it will change much. What we do is certainly more realistic than most couples. Wife-swapping and sexually cheating on a partner, behind their backs, is certainly not a really logical answer. But, I've learned not to question my motives or my actions, just so they bring me the greatest happiness. I want to swing, while I can!

COMMENTS

I find Laura's story revealing that she has not, and might never, get over the shock of discovering her mother with another man. Certainly this is, at least in part, responsible for her seeking out a kind of existence that would not hold her tightly bound to any one man. No doubt she resents her father's lack of real reaction to discovering what his wife was doing behind his back. I had questioned her quite a bit about her father and there was one exchange which was not included in the above.

"Why do you think your father was able to continue to live with your mother after learning about her extramarital relations?"

"I don't think about that. If I were to think about it I guess my conclusions would be he had been weak. I would have divorced a woman who did that to me. If I'd been a man, that is. But of course, I'm a woman, so it doesn't count. I couldn't stand a husband of mine cheating in that manner."

"Yet you sleep with other husbands and you let Jimmy sleep with other women. Isn't that just about the same thing?"

"Not at all." But she seemed nervous, irritated by the question. "I'm not married to Jimmy and if I was, it wouldn't change things. I would still want other men and he would still want other women. So, why get married?"

"What do you think about people like Ann and Ralph? They are married and living with you in a communal manner."

"That's their problem. I really don't think they would have gotten married if they had progressed this far before getting married. See what I mean?"

"Ever wonder why they hadn't gotten divorced?"

"That would be silly, wouldn't it?" She stated this in such a manner that it refused to allow any further comment on the subject.

"Have you ever considered the legal side of what you are doing? It may very well be against the law."

"Living with a man?"

"That and living in a group like you do."

"I don't really believe the law is interested in what we do, just so we don't do it in such a manner that it is made public. We keep our activities behind locked doors, so to speak. We are, on the surface, just a trio of couples sharing expenses, living in a house, rather than renting apartments. Nobody can really stop us from doing that. And from all outward appearances we have our own private bedrooms. As for my living with Jimmy without being married, there are countless of couples living together like that—and those who know or guess don't make it their business. Does *that* answer your question?"

This was a defensive exchange and revealed to me, at least, that Laura is defensive about the way she lives, though she will not admit it to herself or to others. Yet, it seems to be her answer to happiness. Maybe, as she says, it is a more realistic way of living for her.

I was interested in the reasons somebody will live a community-type of sexual life, letting their bodies be used by any member of the community. I wanted to know: What are your reasons, are you happy, and how can you accept such activity in a moral sense?

The answer, as far as Laura is concerned seemed hidden in her childhood, when, after being told a blatant lie by her mother, which as a child she accepted blindly, she discovered her mother to be highly human to the point of cheating on her father. All else, to me, seems rationalization. She will not, while holding her immediate convictions, find a happy home, or enjoy the love of being a mother and having children in the conventional way society accepts. If this is good or bad will depend on what happiness life brings Laura, in the end; and only time and years of it will give this answer.

Talking to the others in her household, I found other answers, other viewpoints, other attitudes, some a little surprising, some conventional.

Jimmy was the next person I interviewed; his story gives a reversal statement as to the real relationship between Laura and the man she has been living with for some years.

CHAPTER TWO

JIMMY

Jim is in his late twenties, working for an electronics firm. He grew up in Los Angeles and served in the army for a time, until he was discharged after an accident that damaged his right leg enough to keep him confined to the hospital for over a year. He is a tall, sandy-haired man with a nervous manner of lighting one cigarette after another; and taking a drag before answering any question. He has strong ideas about life and women and the world in general. He was growing a full beard when I first met him, then finally shaved it off after a couple of weeks, saying it bothered him. He dresses very neatly in well pressed slacks and starched shirts. He has a young, baby-face which will make him the eternal young looking man. A boyish smile plays on his mouth—one that he has learned is highly attractive to women.

When questioned, he would, at times, sit back, consider the point, and then give a thoughtful answer. Many times he would fire the answer back like a bullet, leaning forward, dragging on his cigarette before giving the answer.

[2005 note: While this all happened a number of decades ago, it still stands out as an amazing revelation that fits today's issues. While Jimmy's mention of war and re-

ligion were hitting at things which took place back then, they still, almost frighteningly, apply to today. Our world is split into a major battle between two religious belief systems. The fanatics on both sides claim to be in total all-out conflict. Back then it was more the Cold War after-math of WWII. Then it was the danger of "the bomb" and now it is the danger of terrorism. Many of Jimmy's comments fit today's problems and issues.]

The following is his story, reconstructed from several very long interviews and edited down to its present form.

* * * * * * *

There are several points to make about myself, and maybe I should make them right at the beginning.

I started out in sex a little late in life.

I believed a man should wait until he was married before making it with a woman.

I got all my prudish ideas knocked out of me in the service.

I've always believed that if you have a problem, you should hit at it directly, solve the damned thing and then go on to another problem.

I'm against war, and believe it's time that the United States and the world faces the reality that we're all humans and have a common need for one another. I don't believe in going to church on Sundays, confessing or just getting a spiritual bath, and going out and screwing the world the other six days of the week. If people can't live honestly, with a total sense of morality, they don't have the right to serve or worship a God who is the God of all Churches.

I believe that our bodies enjoy orgasm and should be given a healthy dose of same.

My folks were very religious and I was brought up to believe in their God, but when I reached the age of so-called reason, I developed my own ideas.

I had a sister and she was run over by a car. She was only fifteen, hadn't *lived* life. Maybe that's part of the reason I learned to live *as much as possible!* Life is so damned easily snuffed away. I saw some kids who believed it was sinful to screw before you got married. They marched off and got themselves killed. The accident that got me out of the army killed a good buddy. He'd had a prostitute the night before—his first woman; and last. He hadn't even had a chance to live. Not for me! I want to live in every way, with my guts. We have too short a time in this world.

The first girl I ever had was a whore; heavy, big breasted, in her middle thirties. After being in the army for a couple of months I learned quick. You take pretty much of a beating in basic training and you get to the realization that the world isn't interested in you! If you don't grab what you want in life you might as well put a gun to your head and pull the trigger.

I was lucky; the woman I picked that first time was pretty nice. Like I said, in her middle thirties, running down physically, but a hot sex-pot in bed.

A bunch of us guys from the unit went into town, drank at a bar where we'd been told the girls put out to a guy willing to buy drinks and pay a twenty dollar bill for their services.

I'm not the kind of guy to play around. I might be stubborn as hell about making a move, but when once I've made the decision to move, I'll do it, directly, no holds barred. I'd decided I was going to find out about life and what it was to have a woman. Simple as that.

I drank a lot of beer because I'd learned that makes a hard keep its point up—and a guy having it the first time might just go off too quickly to get a real good shake down for his money.

I danced with this woman, dark hair, long, rolling over her shoulders, big hefty breasts like pillows between us, hips grinding at me like we were screwing right there on the dance floor. We danced with arms about each other, hers around my neck, and mine around her waist. I placed one hand on her soft, generous fanny and kept squeezing. She wasn't about to object to anything sexual. After dancing until both of us were pretty tired, we sat at the small table with the other guys and the three other whores.

Under the table she reached between my legs, unzipped me and fondled my hard penis until it was twitching. Then she replaced her plaything, rezipped my pants, all the time having talked, laughed, and acted as if nothing was happening. I'd been squeezing her leg, having worked her dress up high enough so I could touch the hot flesh of her thigh. After she'd gotten both of us presentable, she turned, smiled at me, said:

"Would you like to leave this place with me now, honey?"

I didn't need a second invitation. She had a small apartment not far from the bar and we walked to it. We never even bothered to turn on the lights. Once the door had been closed she came into my arms and gave me a real deep French kiss, her moist tongue like something hot and alive in my mouth.

After the kiss broke away I asked: "What is this going to cost me?"

She laughed lightly, opened my fly, pulled my hard out and folded her hand about it, real nice and excitingly. "What kind of party do you want, big prick?"

"To be honest, a long one. I have a twenty."

"It'll cost you more than that, if you want a real long one," she murmured, falling to her knees before me, face in front of my stiff erection.

"I want to learn all there is to know about sex, so you tell me what it'll cost." I shuddered to think I had the guts to admit being inexperienced. But I was drunk.

She laughed again. "You're a virgin?"

"I guess you might say that," was my answer. "It'll be twenty, then. I don't get very many virgins as handsome and exciting as you."

And she really meant that! What an amazing break that was for me!

Like I said about this woman, she wasn't young, but she knew her business and I think she really liked sex. In fact she admitted that before she was married she'd been a virgin. Then her husband was killed in the Korean War and she had started picking up men because she needed sex more than most women. She also told me that a girl can get terribly tired of men when she's selling her body every night to a different one; but she also admitted that when something really exciting came along, it was specially good. I think the idea that I was a virgin, and for some reason she found me exciting, made her come on real strong. I'm not kidding myself, or trying to make it sound as if I'm the best lover in the world, or that I was then—because obviously I couldn't have been very good without any experience. But I've heard that experienced women like having a virgin man, just like some guys like seducing a virgin girl.

In any case she covered the end of my penis with her large, generous lips and started lightly sucking and flicking the tip with her tongue. I'd never known that a woman would do such a thing. It was just great! The hot sensations that rocketed through my body were overwhelming.

In moments I was twitching like crazy and she slowly withdrew her lips and stood, lifting her skirt. She led my hand between her legs and I discovered that while she wore garters and stockings there wasn't any panties covering her crotch. She wiggled my finger into her already moist vagina, saying: "Now that's where you put your big prick, love."

She led me through the darkness to a sofa, lay down, drawing me on top of her. We didn't even bother to get undressed. Immediately, she slipped my penis into her vagina, which was firm fitting, moist and so damned soft. The sensations of a first experience in a woman can never be forgotten. They are different from any woman to follow. It's all so new and wonderful. This woman's body burned like fire into my memory and I'll never forget it.

She told me to move slowly in and out, and her own hip motions led the way. Each penetration was more and more exciting. I didn't last more than ten thrusts before I went off like an atomic bomb. She jerked her hips up and down real fast as I started fountaining inside her. As the peak of convulsive climax blew my lights out, she thrust up real hard so I was deeply buried in the moist flesh of her body.

After a while, she led me into the bedroom and we got undressed. Then she went down on me until I was real high, after which she straddled my hips and lowered herself upon the spear of my hard shaft. Her hips moved in circles and then up and down, slowly, torturing me with their actions. The feel of her moist vagina surging around my penis was pure heaven. She rolled her hips around and around, up and down, driving me mad with lusting passion until I couldn't control the constrictions of my penis. She tensed all over, straining, her large breasts thrusting out, a convulsion shuddering through her whole body as we both had a bang-up orgasm together.

We lay next to each other for a long time, then she invited me to start making love to her body, if I wanted to. We kissed and then after a while of being so intimately close, our bodies only lightly touching, though lips and tongues were almost glued against one another. She urged my head down into the large fullness of her huge breasts, moving me back and forth from one to the other. Later she lowered my head towards her stomach, telling me that a woman can get very excited when a man licks his tongue all over her body. I know now that she wanted me to service her swollen pussy, but having already filled her twice with orgasms, and not ever having done such a thing before, I avoided it as if it were a plague. But she got real hot when I started going to town on her stomach and thighs. It was quite an experience. All in all this whore was a very passionate woman, or very good at putting on an act. I must have penetrated her to orgasm half a dozen times that night.

There were a lot of prostitutes in my life during this time, because I didn't know how to go about seducing a girl. But I did learn a lot about sex and prostitutes. Some of them just refuse to kiss a man's lips, some are very cold and business-like, making no attempt to convince you that there should be more to it than in and out, thank you, honey.

Fucking for bucks!

I guess the thing that surprised me the most was the very simplicity of the sex act. No stars, no sudden revelations. Just orgasm inside a woman's cunt or mouth or any place she wants to have you put it.

* * * * * * *

The first orgy I ever experienced was with whores. A couple of buddies wanted to have a real swinging weekend and we all three pooled our money and managed to find three pros willing to ball it for two nights and two days for our bank roll. We only had a few hundred between us, so we made a deal that they'd get all the booze they wanted to drink. Plus whatever cash was left. One girl backed out of the deal but the other two said they knew a young girl who wasn't professional but liked sex a lot, and she would probably be willing to party.

I'd been dating several girls who worked at the base, and one of them was named June. I'd never had the guts to make a pass, because she looked so innocent. She was a little over eighteen, blonde-haired, blue-eyed, and with a build that knocked out just about every guy on the base. I don't know how she had managed to keep a virginal reputation. Though she told me later that she was always willing to get dicked, just so the guys didn't blab all over the place. But in the last months she'd decided it really didn't matter.

Our "orgy" was her second sex party.

I couldn't believe it when she came into the hotel double room we'd rented for the night. She was just as surprised. I felt like a damned fool. But once we were all naked, I found myself with one of the pros and I couldn't keep my eyes off this blonde chick. She went down on one of my buddies like she was a real whore. She went at his dick as if it was a candy cane or something she wanted to devour whole. It's shocking when you learn an innocent girl is screwing like a whore. A bit later grabbed her, really anxious to simply ravish that lovely body. I got her plump breasts, feasting on them. I couldn't get enough of her. She was so hot, so wild. Just one lush chick in head. We balled it like we hadn't had sex for days. We didn't stop until each of us had done a couple of orgiastic tricks.

There's something about an orgy, especially when there's more than one chick there. You can watch the other couples while experiencing orgiastic pleasure with the girl clutching your penis in the fucking hot pussy. You look at the expressions on the other girls' faces and you get excited by that, too. Once, during the first time, four of us were on the bed and the couple next to me was doing a '69', while my chick was straddled over my legs, back to me, pressing my shaft against her sex organ, caressing it with her hands and I started fondling the other girl's nipples, and she screamed out in delight, telling me to really give them a working over, then she continued to work on me, kneeling on all fours. Then my girl lifted up and slipped me into the moist cavity of her hot cunt and began grinding away. I put my free hand around her so it was pawing her large breasts. It was something to be feeling the breasts of two different women at the same time while experiencing intercourse with one of them.

I think this first experience had a lot of effect on me, in many ways. The shock of seeing this one girl I'd thought of as a little virgin prude, and then going into a situation like that one—it was something, really.

* * * * * * *

The next woman, and my first who wasn't a prostitute or acting like a whore at a sex orgy, was the wife of one of the soldiers on the base. I don't really know how it all happened so fast. I didn't expect it at the time, but she taught me something about women and about life that I might not have learned for a long time, if it weren't for her.

Her name, well, we'll just call her Pat.

Pat was in her middle twenties, tall, well built, married to a non-com, and very horny. Her husband, she told me, slept out on her and she had decided a long time before that *what was good for him had to be pretty good for her, too!*

The way it happened was simple enough. I was working at the base laundry and had to make this delivery to her house. It so happened that I made my last delivery there—I was free from then on.

Pat was in a bathing suit that did a lot for her classic figure—a two-piece thing, not quite a bikini, but revealing enough, nonetheless.

It was a hot day and she was sipping a highball. Big dark glasses covered her eyes. She offered me a drink, claiming she felt like talking to somebody.

She was lying on a sundeck and we sat there talking, first about several general topics which I can't remember!

Then she asked if I'd do a favor for her.

"Sure," says I, not guessing what was going to be asked.

She picked up a bottle of suntan cream, extended it to me, asked: "Would you put some of that on my back, I can't reach it and I'm afraid of getting a burn." Her voice was silky, low, like the murmuring of a cat.

Shaken beyond comment, already committed, and painfully aware, by this time, of her most outstanding features, I opened the bottle and put some of the yellowish liquid in the palm of my hand.

She sat up, sorta wiggled her torso, an action that caused her full breasts to bob against the top piece of her bathing suit. Then she slowly dropped the straps of this top piece, slipped her arms free, but being careful to hold the cups in place about her generous breasts.

All this did nothing to help my already excited passions. We were alone and in such a position that nobody could possibly see what we were doing.

The texture of her back, the flesh, so soft and sensual was enough to make any man get ideas and the way she kept turning, looking up into my eyes, making little motions with her shoulders, as if she were feeling a sexual response to the touch left little to my imagination.

"You feel good," she told me quite boldly. "You have a very nice touch."

Any man under such circumstances will find his own desires racing, the need to caress more and more, searching more intimate places to caress. I found my hands automatically reaching around to her side, and a low, soft murmur uttered from her full, half parted lips.

No doubt on purpose, she allowed her hands to relax on the cups of the bathing suit top, an action that gave a good view of her creamy breasts, almost to the rosy nipples. I was already breathing hard, and my third leg was up like a cannon, cocked and ready to shoot.

"You certainly know how to make that exciting to a girl," she told me, turning, lips stopped under mine.

Suddenly it was just too much to take and I was covering her lips with my own. She didn't make any attempt at being modest or coy. Her mouth parted wide, and I felt the probe of her tiny tongue surge out against my teeth, which I parted immediately to this offering. The erotic sensation of that tongue probing deep into my mouth was the spark that fired the explosion. I just couldn't take any more.

My hands slipped under her arms and pushed aside the top of her bathing suit, cupping her full breasts. The nipples were hard dots against the palms of my hand and I worked them in circles, hard, fondling, and squeezing.

She moaned as the kiss broke and her fingers quickly found my pants and just as quickly peeled them down, along with my underpants, until my manhood was totally exposed to her gaze, in all its hard, pulsing glory.

That kind of invitation no man can ever refuse or misunderstand.

I'll never forget her statement at seeing me like that, it burned in my mind like fire.

"Oh, honey, what beautiful meat you have!" Then she was fondling me, like my hands were fondling her breasts. She went on to say something to the effect that she just couldn't get enough of a man's prick and balls. She liked to use such language; a pleased, sensual grin moving her lips as she almost devoured the words. "Oh, honey," she finally said, "get me naked. I want that big wonderful prick in me. I want to feel it squeezed in nice and tight. It's so hard. "

It turned me on, I'll tell you that much. My own hands lowered over her flat belly and tucked under the bottom piece of her bathing suit. Immediately my fingers came in contact with the curly fleece of her pubic area.

She lifted her fanny so I could work off the suit, while at the same time her hands cupped my penis and rubbed it between them, gently, but so sensual that I almost came right there in her hands. I was twitching, I'll tell you that.

She had to release me while I pulled her suit over legs and feet. Then she sat up and started undressing me with caresses that kept me up real big and stiff. She said: "Oh, I just have to do this right. A girl wants it done right. Oh, you…are so large and wonderful! I just love 'em big like that. Big and long and stiff. And so steel hard." She leaned over and kissed my penis, then pulled its tip between her soft moist lips and gently sucked upon it. After that she finished undressing me and then raised her arms up for me. I came down on her like a ton of bricks and she moaned in delight as our sexual organs met, pressing tightly together. We Frenched for a long time, then I was lowering my kisses down to her breasts. She said: "Screw me first, love!"

Her hands gripped my waist and I didn't need any more invitation.

Her legs parted and I felt the moisture of her vagina as the tip of my penis found the entrance to that wonderful moist place of passion.

She jerked up, taking in the full extent of my shaft, then like something insane her hips were grinding away so rapidly, so frantically that I knew it wouldn't last for more than a few moments. She came fast, climaxing in a shuddering cry!

When it was over, she sat up, took my hand and said she wanted to do it again, but in the bedroom.

We embraced for a moment, our bodies flush together, then went into her house. She told me that it had been great but nothing like what was going to follow.

"A girl needs sex just like a man," she explained as we entered her bedroom. "That's the trouble with most men, they think a woman doesn't want sex the same way. It took me a long time before I was able to screw a man without being afraid of shocking him. How wonderful it is to be yourself. *If boys just knew how a girl felt!* I grew up in a so-called respectable family and nobody talked about sex, but I learned fast and found how difficult it is for a girl to get her signals across to most guys. They think she is fast or cheap if she wants to get a sexual thrill. I'll tell you one thing: don't ever make the mistake that a girl doesn't want a man's prick sticking in her cunt. She wants it just like a man, but she can't come right out and say it. She will play it cool, sometimes even refusing to be kissed. Believe me, that's a sure sign a girl wants it, because she is frightened the boy will start things and never finish."

We sat on the bed, facing each other, legs parted, so our sexual organs were exposed to one another. She reached out and started fondling my penis while talking. "I just love to play with a lovely cock like this. It's fun to see a man's prick grow from something small to something big and swollen and hard, knowing you're causing that to happen. I used to want to reach down between some of my dates' legs and as them to just give me a piece of your meat, honey. Some guys can be really stupid about girls."

She told me how a girl will play cold, but that she won't ever go out with a man she isn't sexually interested in. She put it something like this: "A boy and girl meet and they either find each other sexually attractive or they don't date. A boy gets excited about a girl's body and so he asks her out. What is he really interested in? Even if he doesn't admit it? He wants to put his prick inside her cunt. He wants to screw her. What do you think a girl really wants? She wants the same thing. But society makes it almost impossible for her to get this big thrill without looking like a whore."

By that time she was so overwhelmed that she took my hand, put it on her pussy, said: "Pump your finger in me, and around the entrance, honey, and I'll do a few tricks with your oh so lovely prick!"

I did exactly as she said while her own fingers were playing with my erection and balls, making such erotic sensations to tingle through me that I was jerking faster and faster with my finger as she kept caressing and jerking me to orgasm. Afterwards she said: "That's fun, watching the expression on a man's face when I'm doing something like this."

* * * * * * *

I guess every man has to learn about sex and about women the hard way—or, maybe it's really the beautiful way. I can say one thing, from then on I didn't go after prostitutes, because I'd learned that a woman who gives of herself, because she honestly wants sex with you, is far better than a woman who sells herself to you because it is her way of making a living.

I get all choked up about how wives are supposed to be nothing but legalized prostitutes. Anybody who has had it with a whore and then with a woman who gives of herself, both physically and emotionally, will know that a wife is far from a legalized prostitute. Oh, sure there are women who get married who really don't like sex, or think they don't like it. Well, as far as I'm concerned, that's their hang-up and certainly their husband's. I've found that if you make certain demands on a woman, right from the beginning, you don't have any problems about the sex thing. And, in the first place, a man shouldn't be foolish enough to get tangled up with a woman who doesn't meet his sexual needs as a total partner.

I've known guys who get married simply because they want sex with a girl. I wouldn't marry a woman I hadn't slept with first! These same guys who get all screwed up in marriage, because they waited until the marriage ceremony before balling it with the "little woman" will say *I'm* the crazy one. They claim that any girl who will put out to a man, without being married to him, is something short of a cheap tramp. I guess the girls they married, in some cases, that is, would be just that if they let themselves be screwed before getting married, because that is what they would think of themselves.

I can't help thinking it's all backwards. Take Laura. She's not afraid to admit she likes sex, for sex and nothing more. But she also likes to be loved. There's a complete difference between love and sex—not that they can't go hand in hand. And, certainly, sex is far more important as an emotional thing when there's a feeling of affection between you and the woman.

Orgasm is just fine. There's nothing like a woman getting down on her knees before you, like some sex-slave, putting her lips around your cock and sucking away. It's just great. It feels terrific to you, her moist, warm mouth tugging, her tongue licking away—sure it feels great! But is the girl getting something out of it? Maybe. And I mean that *maybe* very strong. A whore is doing what she is being paid to do, a woman who is really turned on sexually might do such a thing because she's just crazy with passion and just wild about the fact that your cock can give such orgiastic pleasure to her, no matter where she lets you place it. That's the difference.

Laura goes ape with a man she cares about, and she can be pretty wild even with a guy she hardly knows.

I think that's the most important thing.

This army base wife had come onto me strong and taught me that a woman can really enjoy sex, simply because she likes it so much. She can enjoy it even with a stranger, just because suddenly something physical has happened and it seems right.

You know, I've talked to guys who would turn down a piece of ass, simply because they think it is wrong to screw a nice girl! I personally think it's wrong to turn down any woman.

I remember one woman, she was about ten years older than me, who said: "Jimmy, when a woman gives—offers herself to you—she is giving the greatest gift possible. When the man turns her down, it is a great ego blow. She has offered herself, offered to give of her body, a very great gift of love—even if it is only a sexual love. To have such a gift turned down is a terrible blow. What greater offering can a woman make other than her whole self, physically...and emotionally. And don't ever get the idea that *any* woman can allow her body to be invaded by a man, without having some emotional reactions. It is what makes up a woman. Even if it's purely sexual there will be emotional reactions, if only on a subconscious level. Don't make her think she is undesirable. Tell her some lie. But one that makes some logical sense. Let her cling to something other than the idea she has been rejected. It will still hurt her, but it won't be quite so shattering; it will be easier to laugh it off."

I'd been carrying on quite an affair with that woman, and she taught me something important about life. I really don't want to go into the details of that affair, other than to say she was a divorced woman who had been dumped for a younger girl. She told me a lot about how a woman feels under such conditions. I learned. Later, too, that people who go through a divorce will, most of the time, seek out a series of affairs to prove to themselves that they are desirable to the opposite sex. I guess it's especially true of men, because they seem to have such a great ego about the sex thing; but women react the same way, to some degree, depending on what kind of person they are. Social conditioning alters our actions. But they, on a basic, animalistic level, have the same desire to prove to themselves they are wanted, loveable and desired by the opposite sex.

I was lucky to learn something about the way women think, at an early age, because I had a few good breaks.

On the surface, I guess, that would make one wonder

why I have fallen into this group thing. To me it is a very logical way to live, because we are all honest about ourselves and about our sexual urges. There aren't any real lies about how one feels about the other. I started living with Laura because there was an emotional basis for this. We care about one another, but not to the degree where we want to smother one another. Well, maybe I should put that another way: we care enough for the other not to be overly possessive. That can crush real feelings. Being held too tight is damaging to the soul.

I respect Laura and I understand her to some extent. She's a woman who wants love and orgasm in a big way. To me, it's amazing that two people can meet and share one another in the way we share one another, and be so damned happy.

When I got out of the service, I wanted to swing, to live a little, to learn what life was all about in every way.

I was a little bitter about the world situation and how we have to live with the bomb and how the government is run by people who don't really understand the needs and desires of the people. They're of the old generation with old fashioned ideas about world politics. They think force will get what they want, where I believe open-minded love will. Love everybody as you would love yourself and people will start living in peace. All these young men getting killed; hell, it doesn't matter where the wars are being fought, they are there and people are getting killed *for nothing*!

And, as far as I'm concerned, we have enough problems right here in America. The Negro situation is inane. What the hell's wrong with letting people have a chance to live a good life? What right do we whites have to say they aren't equal to us; just because their skin is black? Hell, we're fighting a war for people with yellow skins. What insanity causes such foolish reasoning?

Well, I've learned something about myself. I grew up

with old fashioned ideas about women and sex, and I learned it was all in the wrong bag. Like Laura might say: I was bombed out to learn the truth.

The same reasoning has been used to say women shouldn't have sexual freedom. Women are supposed to be possessions. Hell and crap. I don't think a woman is a possession any more than I am her possession. We give of each other freely, because that's what we want, not because some magic religious words have been said over us and made us man and wife. First of all, marriage takes place in the mind, and if it isn't here, it doesn't exist, no matter what law or a man might claim.

It might seem all this has nothing to do with my way of living, because there are many married couples who believe the same way I do, but are totally loyal to one another. Yet it has a lot to do with my attitude about life and the social structure of our nation.

Sex is a very important part of everybody's life. Why deny the desire to screw a woman? Well, to be truthful it is more than screw, and I must admit that I really don't think of it in the sense of "screwing the world" or "screw you, you bastard," but more like the act of sexual intercourse, of making love, can all be wadded up into one word: Screwing. Loving. Sexing it. Making it. But it's more than that. Loving the world. Making it in life, in every way. Having sex with women, because you enjoy it, because the woman enjoys it.

Why lie to myself. I like orgasm and I like feeling the difference between one woman's pussy and another woman's.

Sure, in the end, it's all the same. You have orgasm. And in the end all you're thinking about is that wonderful orgiastic sensation.

But when I make love to Laura, it is something else. Or even when I make love to Ann or Nancy, it is different.

Let me tell it this way.

Laura and I will climb into bed together, naked, pressing our bodies close, feeling the texture of one another, thrilling to the softness and hotness and warmth of our caring about one another.

I might say something like: "Oh, Laura, I love you." She might say the same thing to me. But our whole bodies are saying that in the first tender touches. I find myself caressing her soft, yielding flesh, wanting to make her feel the emotion that is welling up in me. I feel tenderness, warmth, a wanting to clutch to her flesh, a wanting to protect her from any physical or emotional harm. I feel this love welling up inside me so fantastically that it overwhelms all other considerations. And in this I simply mean, I'm not screwing some broad or having some broad screw me, but I'm making love in the most spiritual sense of the word. I can't control the physical and emotional desires that finally cause my hands to cup over her breasts, to feel her nipples harden, to finally kiss them with lips and tongue. I want her to feel my love in the tenderness of my fullest feelings.

And when I end up doing something like putting my lips between her legs, kissing the depth of her sexual organ and finally press myself deep within her body, in the final acts of our love-making, it's something more than merely physical sexual outlet. I thrill to the fact that it is her flesh tugging on my penis, that it is her body responding to my penetrations.

But with one of the other girls I can sometimes feel a sense of affection almost as deep, because I know them, care about them, and I thrill to the fact that they are responding to my body, my thrusts of passion that is entering their total being.

Yet there is a lot more than this kind of love, believe me. That's the beauty of our kind of living. We all share the same goals, to some extent, because we are working for the same thing: survival of the whole. We care about one another, live together like some kind of completely united family.

When an orgy takes place, then you really have something going.

I remember with great pleasure the times when we'll be in the darkness together on two double beds that have been placed side by side, hooked tightly by belts. The room is dark and we're all naked and you reach out and try to discover who you are touching. You feel a soft breast, yielding under your fingers and hear a moan of pleasure. Then some tiny hand searches out to discover your hard penis, starts caressing...or maybe it might be some girl's lips. You might find yourself kissing a girl's cunt, while another is giving you a blow job, or you might be penetrating one girl while another is Frenching your mouth, while you finger another's breasts.

I remember the first time I took on Ann and Nancy, alone. Everybody else was out of the house, working or shopping, and I felt the urge to have a sex party, and as Ann passed me, she was wearing shorts and a loose fitting blouse, I grabbed her thigh, pulled her close, ran my hand into her blouse and felt warm, soft naked flesh. She wasn't wearing a bra and the feel of her sent me wild.

She looked at me, then came into my arms with a little delighted moan of pleasure, a smile of delight working her soft lips. We kissed real passionately while I fondled her lovely tiny breast, my other hand between her legs, where she held my fingers in place against her thighs.

There's something real sexy about grabbing a girl, running your hand into her blouse and finding naked flesh. She dug this too, and we really came on strong together.

Nancy happened to enter the living room at that time and giggling with delight, came over, knelt down and placed her hand on my fly, unzipping it and started almost immediately to use her mouth in a way that was not meant to turn me off.

I kept kissing Ann, while pulling her blouse off, then working her shorts down, while Nancy went to town on me.

This kind of double stimulation can be pretty wild. You sorta let yourself go, sensually. You feel the softness of two women at once. You become aware of their sexual responses to you as a man. There's nothing like making it with a woman you care about, and when you double the take—letting your body and sexual acts stimulate two women at once, that makes it even better.

I know that some people would think such attitudes and acts as perverse, against Nature.

Well, I don't believe that sex is just for having babies. In fact, maybe they should outlaw the whole concept of sex and babies being one and the same. Sex should be for pleasure. There are too many people who rationalize. They like sex, but they tell themselves it's natural to have babies, and unnatural to think of the sex act simply as something that gives physical pleasure.

I feel sorry for such soft-heads. And that's what they are! They're not thinking. They're reacting to total conditioning given from birth on.

We're facing a terrible problem in the world today. If people don't start acting intelligent, realizing that overpopulation is facing the world, that we just might overpopulate ourselves out of existence—life is going to be damned hellish.

You know, I've thought about this a lot. The world of tomorrow. And I believe the kind of life we have—our group—is in a way expressing the future, *today*!

Well, the way things are going on now, when couples get married and have half a dozen children, reproducing like damned stupid rabbits, we're going to end up in huge monster apartment houses, sharing rooms with other couples. There won't be anything like owning a home, having a piece of land you can call your own. You'll live in combines; one apartment...maybe three rooms, with three or four other couples. There won't be any privacy for sexual acts. It will be impossible to get any intimacy in a totally personal, private way with *one* person. Living together like that, smelling the sweat and sex of other couples, knowing what's going on behind a drawn curtain, hearing the sounds of love, the passions, the rhythms, it's going to be natural that you'll start wondering about some of the other people you're living with. Sex *will* become communal. It *has* to, when you have people living together in a tight little spaces.

We live in a fairly plush house, one none of us could afford alone. We have plenty of room to keep our sex lives private, but we realize it wouldn't really be realistic in an emotional way.

Look at some of the problems we solve.

If a couple gets mad, the man wants to screw some other gal; hell, all he has to do is go to one of the other girls in the house and they bang it up, and they get a lot of frustrations off their minds. They learn to interrelate on a far greater level.

But forgetting that for a moment.

We've talked about the future. In this, I mean, the future that faces all of us and the children being born. We believe that couples should have a greater freedom in sexual expression, for emotional health reasons, but *not* with the idea of having babies.

There should be a few laws made to control birth rates, before it's too late.

One might be: If a person is dying from illness or accident, and medical science can save their lives, then they should be healed, but at the cost of fixing them so they can't have any more children. Cruel? Sure it is! But what if science hadn't been able to save their lives? The possible future generations wouldn't have followed. We'd be saving a life, but saying in effect: The price is no more children from a person who has almost had both feet in the grave. Hellishly cruel. But it is far crueler to allow more children to be brought into the world and cause a dangerous problem in over-population.

Another way would be: Couples can't have more than two children! After two kids, they are sterilized—or any pregnancy would be aborted. That alone would cut the population down. I don't know how much, but figuring that there is a certain amount of death rate before age of reproduction and then there are those couples who either wouldn't have any children or no more than one—we'd more than halve the human race in a generation...or so. Cruel? Sure, but what other choice do we have? Over-population!

Nothing makes me madder than these rabbit couples who think sex is for having babies and they have as many as they can. Usually they are stupid, uneducated, and poor. Sadly enough the rich and intelligent limit, plan their families on a scale they can afford.

So, I keep saying, those who want to cast stones at our way of living together on a community basis, better take a closer look at what *they* are responsible for by their narrow, damned stupid ways and attitudes.

Maybe none of this has anything to do with my attitude about sexual freedom of expression.

Maybe I'm rationalizing. But I believe it's a far more healthy rationalization.

We are seeing the future, the way it should be, but not the way it will be if things continue as they have up until now.

We are living together in luxury. We have an inter-relationship that is meaningful.

Like that day that both Ann and Nancy were going to town with me. They discovered I wanted some action and they went along with it. They wanted to give and wanted to get some of the action themselves.

We've talked about that, too. Nothing phony about our attitudes. The girls have openly admitted that they found it exciting and interesting to have more than one lover. I believe it was Ann that told me: "Why be limited to one penis. Sometimes I wish I could have all three of you at once. Yet there is a difference between all three of you men. I find it wonderful. I'm not afraid to experiment, and through that experimentation I learn something about myself and other people."

One thing I hope will be made very clear: The world is phony, has a lot of damned stupid rules that don't make sense, if you look at them honestly. People dig people. You can be attracted to more than one woman and you can want to make it with her. Not that you want to screw every woman you meet. But it's damned nice to know there are a few there who can respond and relate to you on a personal level.

With the world so screwed up, what right does anybody have to point a finger at us and say we're wrong? War is wrong! Killing is wrong. Tell me this: why should sex be considered wrong when war is condoned?

Hell, I know all this sounds unimportant, considering what the message of this whole thing is supposed to be. But you can't split sex from the manner in which a man— or woman, for that matter—thinks about life.

I'd rather beat a girl's ass to...well, that's another bit.

I've never stopped being surprised about women. Take Ann, for instance. One time she was furious at Ralph and had come to me, in the living room, blouse open, tits sticking out, her skirt unzipped. I was watching television, the others were screwing in my bedroom—that is, Laura was with another couple. Ann grabbed my arm, said, "Come with me, lover."

We went into the den, closed the door and then she pulled down her skirt, stepped out of her panties, slipped off her blouse and then instructed me to sit on the sofa.

Then she lay across my lap and said, "Hit me, real hard, love."

That one shocked me some, because I'd never done anything like that before. They'd been living with us for only a few weeks, and there had been no reason to discover Ann's desire to be spanked.

I lightly tapped her fanny, and she wiggled, said to hit her harder. I did it a little harder and her fanny quivered. "Harder, love, as hard as you can!" she demanded, gripping the sofa in an effort to prepare herself.

So I hit her, pretty hard, and she moaned in delight, pleading for even a harder hit. Getting the message, I started really smacking her fanny until she was sobbing in pain and pleasure. I kept this up for some time, until her fanny was red-hot looking. She was quivering and choking, clawing at the sofa. Suddenly she sobbed, "enough!" and came up into my arms, covering my face with voluptuous kisses. Her right hand raced down between my legs, unzipped my fly and started fondling greedily away. Before I realized it, she had straddled me and was fairly hammering up and down on my lap, her tongue thrusting deep into my mouth in rhythm with the thrust of her hips. It was some session. Her pussy was moist and hot from the first penetration and she continued until both of us had come several times.

Afterwards, as we were smoking, she said: "I guess you are pretty surprised about this thing. But I like a good spanking when Ralph and me have a fight. I don't know, but maybe I'm trying to punish myself for being angry at him, hating him. Maybe it's something about guilt. I just don't know! But I just love to be spanked and spanked to orgasm."

What do you do to a girl like that? It's interesting that she was able to guess the real reason for her need. Or at least a reason that has seemed logical enough, I guess.

There are a lot of things that go on at the house. You

have to understand a basic thing about all of us. We admit that sex is fun. We admit that we like sexing it with each other, and we know that sex can be a fine outlet for emotional problems.

That's really the most important part of it all.

Nancy came home from work at the bank one afternoon, almost in tears because she has a bastard department head. I just don't understand what the hell makes companies pick hard bastards to run rod over other people. They seem to think the hard-nosed bastard makes the best section head. I've learned, in my own experience in life, and from talking to others, that the way to handle people is to show respect to them, to try to help, not control and dictate to them. This son-of-a-bitch had gotten Nancy aside and told her she was out too many times, that she couldn't be out of work any more without being fired. She told me it wasn't what he said, but the way he was saying it. Cold eyes, the look of a man who doesn't believe people get sick. She said it this way: "We all, the girls at the bank, have talked about it, and they all say the same thing. When they have called in or their husbands have called in, saying they are sick and can't go to work that day, this SOB acts like you're telling him a lie. He'll say, "Yes," like he's saying, "go right ahead, tell me another lie!" He fired a girl who was working part time, simply because she didn't want to work full time. They had hired her on the promise of giving her a part time job."

I've been in situations much like this one. One guy I worked under was easy going. If you made a mistake he respected you, explained the problem and then knew you felt like hell without being bawled out. The man who replaced him would climb all over you for the smallest mistake. One fellow who was considered just about the best worker at the place, went all to pieces and started making mistakes all over the place, just because this bastard was riding his back. When they had just about fired or released everybody, other than the new boss, they finally realized who was to blame, but too late.

You know, most companies would rather fire every employee than the section head?

So what's that have to do with our kind of living together? Well, Nancy felt so damned hurt and bitchy that it was obvious that the only way to get her mind off it was to have a real crazy sex party. So the three of us guys got her in the bedroom and started giving her a real physical and sexual working over. She went crazy with passion and lust. She blew Dave, while fondling Ralph like crazy and let me possess her vagina. Then we'd take turns loving her, or she'd have us stand in a circle around her and she'd start doing all kinds of crazy things to our bodies. The thing I'm trying to say is that she needed a real spree, a complete blackout and we gave it to her. Laura was having her period and Ann kept her company while we did our best to blow Nancy's emotional fury through orgasm. A total, complete, emotional, and physical blast-out orgasm.

It took the three of us to do it. But Nancy was a much more happy woman by the end of that night session.

That's the thing, too. With more than one person, there is somebody willing to cooperate, even if they don't really feel like it.

Once I came home, depressed, and Laura just wasn't in the mood for anything intimate. Ann and Nancy flipped a coin, Nancy ending up as my partner and we went into her room and she really gave me a sex party, even though she wasn't too much in the mood. But we have this working arrangement *to help each of us.* If we need it somebody has to serve as a partner.

I've been tired myself, but more than willing to return a favor to one of the girls, if they needed something to help them over some emotional hump. Maybe they simply want to be pressed in between two guys. Or maybe they wanted simply to be loved, like a lovely woman, desired and understood and wanted. Just held.

When you have only one mate, it is pretty hard to make a good balance. When there are more than one to pick from there's always somebody to give you a helping hand.

Funny thing, later, after that time I learned how fun it can be to spank a girl, I learned that Laura, also, liked this kind of thing. We all talked some about it and we've done some exploration in such matters, but generally there is only a limited experimentation of this kind.

After all, how far does one want to go? I really don't know the answer for most people, but for us, well, we don't live on sex all the time!

I don't want you to get the idea it's all sexual orgies. We're like any other group of people, everybody has their own hang-ups and their own sexual needs, but there are other needs.

Like going to movies; getting involved with certain activities. Like the Civil Rights thing. We haven't done anything active on that level, but we've certainly talked up a storm. Between ourselves and others. Generally we don't like getting involved with other people or outside problems, if you understand. Not in an active way. We have enough involvement within our own little circle of friends.

That's the whole bit, though, in a way. That's the reason we function as we do. We rebel and reject the attitudes of the older generation. Where does one get off saying that because a person's skin is black, green or yellow that they are not equal with you?

Take Germany during World War Two. They were crazy in the head to march off all the Jews to camps and kill them off. There could have been a much better solution: Send them to the front lines, let them fight for the Fatherland, because they believed and thought of themselves as Germans who just happened to be Jewish by religious faith.

Horrid idea? Sure. But what really happened was far worse. They died without dignity.

But the interesting thing is, how many Jews hate Germans, now they turn and spit on the German face—while at the same time screaming, crying like babies, that everybody is against the Jews. I'd say the best way for somebody to be loved, really loved and understood and respected, is to love, understand and respect others. If you hate, you'll get hate. And all these books that keep screaming about the Germans and the Second World War can be counterproductive in the long run. Can't people forget the past and live in the Now and present, looking forward to the future? Oh, sure, we should remember the lessons of the past. But to keep harping on them. The Germans of today are a different people. Most of them were children when the war was on. They're paying taxes out of their pockets to pay for a war they had nothing to do with. Sure, we can say they are lucky not to be slaves to the United States, France and Great Britain. But that's not the way of the world today. Not the American way, anyhow! But it all goes back to closed minds. Hate Jews. Hate Germans. Hate Japs. Hate Negroes. Hate sex.

If there's anything we should hate, it's hating hatred and people who hate. And that's part of the reason we, or at least *I,* believe that people should find their own form of love and their own way of expression and make the most of their lives.

We have a love group, one that interrelates in a total way. We express ourselves totally. We give to one another as selflessly as possible. We think of ourselves as one big happy family.

If I say something like, I really screwed her hot cunt with my hot prick, I don't mean that in a dirty or nasty way. I think it would sound false to say I made love to her thing with my thing; or had sexual intercourse with her sexual organ.

It's love, and it's love to say the basic words that can excite another. It excites me when one of the girls come up and say, Jimmy fuck me with your hot prick. Or stick my pussy with your cock. Or I'm hot, love: I want that big meat of yours feeding my love-nest. All that is expressing sexual desires in a sexual, raw, basic way, meant to communicate a sexual directive. The girl is hot, she wants sex and she wants you to feel her heat, immediately and wants you to know in basic, earthy gut-terms exactly how she feels and what she wants. Cock-fucking her pussy.

And again, I get back to one basic thing: it's better to use four letter words than to go out and take a gun and kill a President. Or to kill some slat-eyed slob in South Vietnam. It's better to screw a pussy with your hot cock than to cock a gun and murder somebody. That's the trouble with our world today: people just won't go out and get what they really want, they hang themselves up emotionally and take it out on the wrong guy.

Kill, don't fuck. That's the basic cry!

What's life all about? Tell me that? For war? To have millions of dollars? To overpopulate the world? To hate?

Hell no! *I think it's to love life and make the most out of your existence.*

Like I said, I have a hang-up against society and the blasted phonies that are driving us down the path to mutual destruction. Take television and movies and the newspapers, anything. People would rather talk and see violence spread out all around them than to see two healthy young people making love. Hell, screwing. Just fucking their brains out.

Now you tell *me* who is crazy?

Is it better to kill or is it better to love?

Sure, I want my sex to be private. And I mean this in the following way: Private between me and whoever else is entering the scene—no matter how many. If two girls get a charge sharing my body between them, hell, what's wrong with that? If I don't mind sharing one girl with another or several other guys and that's what she wants, why shouldn't we? Who is hurt?

An interesting statement on life, I believe, is that a man can be gassed for raping a girl, but be given only life for killing somebody and then get out after a few years because they've been a good little person.

Most women who have been raped have survived the experience. Nancy can tell you something about that. We've talked that over quite a bit. She was raped. She survived. It would seem insanity to kill the person who raped her. But, put the guy away for life and correct his sexual hang-up—or simply fix him so he can't have any more sexual feelings. But kill him? That's the right of the father or brother or husband, *only* in an automatic reaction of passion. I could see myself killing somebody who might rape Laura, because it would be an act of passionate fury, but I don't believe I should be able to get away with it, legally.

The thing is, when you have a phony world like this one, living on the edge of Atomic destruction warring for no really honestly sane reason, over-populating itself out of existence, then saying sexual freedom is something bad or perverted, only a man out of his nut could possibly believe what we do is wrong.

In simple terms, if I want to have a sex with a girl, and she wants it, too, and she's part of the family, why not?

But, don't kid yourself, we have our own set of morality. And I'll admit, that's a little bit fantastic, too. It shows how we are still products of our society, that we can't take the complete yoke off—that we are conditioned. But my feeling is that our morality and restrictions are at least more realistic and more honest. We don't go out seducing young virgins or picking people up for kicks: we keep it in the family. Oh, we'll have parties with other people who believe the same way we do, but that's something else, completely. That's a get-together. Everybody has parties and ours just go a step further, that's all. We don't play the phony scene; that's all.

But please quote me on this: If you're honest with yourself, you have to admit there are more than one or two people you'd like to have sexual intercourse with. So, why hang-up the stick with one girl? Why not live a more realistic life? Why not get together with other couples you like, share a nice expensive home. Share sexual experiences and love. But don't go out and cheat on each other, behind each other's backs.

Don't be a phony.

COMMENTS

The anger and fury of some of Jimmy's words and statements were always expressed by his getting up and pacing the floor, striking out at the air, as if he were hitting something or someone. I have known a lot of people with a lot of frustrations and angers, but Jimmy was violent to a highly emotional sense about what he believed in and what he hated. Yet, his ideas, while not all right, were not unfounded. The world is in many ways phony and *the young people are repulsed by this.* But they are phony, too.

I asked him at one time about his attitudes about sleeping with a Negro woman.

He looked up at me, his face suddenly becoming very serious, almost withdrawn.

"You know, I've never really thought of it—like *really* doing it! Oh, there have been some who were highly attractive and even sexy, but I never actually thought: why not make it with her!"

I asked him why and he said: "Well, to be truthful I just don't know."

"Would you sleep with a woman, a very beautiful one, let's say, who made it clear she was willing to have intercourse with you?"

"I don't know, come to think of it." He sounded as amazed as his statement was surprising.

"Well, I'll put it this way, could you perform cunnilingus on her?"

He made a quick face, then controlled his response, said: "Funny how we are conditioned. Our minds say one thing, our emotions say another. I guess, under the right conditions I might, if I was hard up enough. But the idea is not really the most attractive one."

"You are just as bad as those you hate so much," I pointed out with some humor.

"No I'm not!" Jimmy disagreed. "For one; I admit I'm wrong, that this attitude is wrong. I shouldn't feel any difference, and maybe I wouldn't if the situation presented itself. And for another; there are a lot of bastards who would relish making it with a Negro woman, because they have some idea that sex is dirty and they are out to have some kind of dirty thrill. They aren't making love to the woman or to her body, but raping or defiling the woman for psychological reasons of their own. Hell, such a white man would be getting a double thrill *because* the woman was black. No. There's quite a difference. At least I believe there is."

I had to agree with Jimmy on that point. What seemed interesting to me was the fact that he was honest enough to admit his reluctance to accept the idea of interracial sexual intercourse, especially because I had asked this question about the time he was so angrily shouting down those who have blind hatred for blacks. Because of that, one can easily come to the conclusion that Jimmy honestly expressed his feelings and attitudes, leaving little out.

He did say, a few moments later, on this subject: "Really, there shouldn't be any reservation in my mind. I should be able to look at the idea of sexual relations with a red, white, yellow, back, blue, green, you name it, woman without any hesitation! It should only depend on the human being under the skin—not the color that masks the body. But I didn't claim to have all the answers, or that I was perfect or that our *way* is perfect. I just simply believe out way is a better way, a more honest one. At least we're trying. And that's a start!"

CHAPTER THREE

NANCY

"Sure I was raped. And it's not a very nice thing to happen to a fourteen-year-old girl, no matter how it happened. I really don't like to talk about it, but I've learned how to do so. You have to face yourself honestly and not be afraid to examine any experience, no matter how bad it might be."

I had asked her, first thing, about the rape, because I was interested in following through with this experience of hers and seeing how it might have affected her later attitudes about sex. She is the kind of woman who makes one believe there is nothing that might shock her. She is maturely developed and highly attractive with a large, sensual mouth.

As the following dialogue will show, Nancy believes she is a woman well adjusted, even though her early experiences in sex were bitterly cruel and unjust.

I guess it would be best to tell you something about my family, then maybe it will be understood why it was such a shock...being raped. It's pretty bad for any girl, but it can be terrible when you've been very much protected. I was overly protected and my folks thought that a nice girl didn't have sex until she was married, even rape was sinful.

We were a close family, in the beginning. I remember having some wonderful times at home, as a child. But things changed very rapidly. Rape changes things for a girl, no matter what. She suddenly learns about sex and something of the sordid side of life. It's a terrible experience, even at best. But when you have parents who react like my folks did, forget it.

I guess it's a terrible thing to say, but the folks were real bastards. I'll never understand how they could act like they did. Both were highly religious. Can you imagine blaming a girl for being raped. Yet that's exactly what they did.

Up until I was fourteen, everything was just fine. The folks were understanding toward me, in that they tried to make things as easy as possible for a young girl growing into maturity. I was told that there were two kinds of girls: those who would go to Heaven, because they lived sinless lives and those who went to Hell. I *was* told that a nice girl would not let a man or boy touch her, even for a kiss until she was engaged, and would never have relations with anybody until she is married.

I learned that it felt good to touch myself between the legs. I learned how it felt to run my finger along the fleshy area about my vagina. I learned, in short, how to masturbate. And I liked it but didn't quite believe it was sinful until one evening Mom walked into the bathroom, when I was standing in front of the wall mirror, naked, caressing my young breasts and fingering my flushed vagina.

Boy, was she *shocked*. I can't remember all the things she said, but they were blunt enough. They went something like this, though: "You're a dirty, sinful little girl! You will go to Hell for doing that!" She went on like that for a long time and Dad heard and when he came in and saw what was going on, he grabbed hold of me, sat down on the john and turned me over his knees, smacking my fanny until anguished tears were streaming down my cheeks. I'd never seen him so furious.

They gave me a long lecture about the sins of masturbating and said that if I ever did a thing like that again I would really wish I'd never been born. They made me confess my sins over the Bible and made me promise never to do such a thing again as long as I lived.

That night changed my whole attitude about them and life. But it was only the beginning.

When I think back about it, I find it difficult to believe they could be so damned old fashioned and dumb. How can people think like that in the twentieth century? But, then, I guess they aren't so much to blame as *their* parents, who conditioned them against sex. I would imagine they confessed to sins for making love to one another. No, maybe not. But I guess it's hard for most people to think of their folks having sexual intercourse. That's one thing that got to Laura—but she saw something totally different. I think, funny though it might seem, that I would have been delighted to walk into my mother's bedroom and discover she was screwing a man, *any* man!

Interesting how people are different. Laura was really hung up on that for a long time. But maybe you can't blame her.

What happened to me was really quite simple. My folks never quite believed me. But they were pretty unrealistic in every way, concerning sex, that is. Until Mother walked in and saw me playing with myself, we had a fairly good relationship. In fact, I think, Mother tried to make things better, but it was too late, by then. It was very shortly after that discovery that I was raped. Dad still thought of me as being very sinful. Oh, what a damned fool *he* was! And it took me a long time to get over the shock of everything. And I mean *everything*! I know I never liked my parents much after that discovery in the bathroom; though I didn't admit it until after the rape.

Rape is terrible. Some women it shatters for life. Some

can pass it over fairly casually. Some, like me, have to take time.

It was late afternoon and I'd been visiting a girl friend. Probably I shouldn't have done that without letting the folks know about it.

Nonetheless, I started home when the sun was just going down. It was quite a walk and I was a little tired, so when this car pulled up to the side of the curb and a man in his late forties, I would imagine, leaned out the window and asked if I wanted a ride, I did a very foolish thing—I accepted, on impulse.

Now the folks had warned me about such things, but I'd also heard from kids at school that they sometimes hitched a ride and nothing terrible had ever happened. In fact, this man sure looked nice. Very friendly and almost fatherly. He didn't seem the kind of man who was degenerate. But, that just goes to show you how wrong you can be.

The minute I got into the car and we pulled into traffic, he started saying things like: "A girl like you shouldn't be out alone so late. You never know what might happen. There are a lot of people who might get the wrong idea. Now you take me, for one. How do you know I might not have the idea we could do something together? I might have picked you up for some fun. After all, most girls won't let a strange man pick them up."

It was a strange conversation, but I didn't feel alarmed, really, until he turned off the main highway, in the wrong direction. I mean, the wrong direction to get me home. I told him that I'd better get out, because I lived a few blocks up the other road.

He laughed at me, then.

I said something to the effect I didn't think it was very funny, and would he please let me out.

The guy turned, reached out and fondled my leg, high up. "You are really a very beautiful young girl. And no girl your age would get into a car with a strange man, unless she wanted something."

I got frantic, frightened and pleaded with him to let me out. He laughed, mocking me.

I started to reach for the door handle, desperate enough to leap out of the moving car.

What happened then was so startling that I couldn't believe it.

His right hand slammed across my face, real hard. It was such a stunning blow that I almost lost consciousness. I became aware of his doing something with my hands and arms, but was too dazed to quite understand what or resist. When total awareness returned I found myself handcuffed. At first I thought he must be some cop or something. But that wasn't it at all.

I'll be quite honest, if that's possible. I was scared to death. But I've had a lot of time to think things out and I have to face one fact: In the end, there was something very exciting about what happened. I didn't accept this for years, though I understand it now. I did climax. I did have orgasm because my body is highly sexed, I know that now, and it did respond to the rape. But rape was a long way away at that moment.

I pleaded with him, but he just laughed, saying that if I didn't shut up, he'd club me across the face again. There just wasn't anything I could do. So I remained silent. And frightened! And I'll tell you one thing, it *is* a frightening experience. It would be for a *woman,* because you don't know if you'll come out of such a thing alive. To a kid, it's even more terrifying. You don't have any idea about sex, though you know something horrible is going to happen. He drove me out of town and then took a side road until he came to a small wooded area. There he parked the car and pulled me out of it.

I struggled at first, but he laughed, hit me real hard. The thing that amazes me to this day is that he didn't kill me. It was one of those lucky things; maybe he might have if the mood had been different.

The next thing I knew was that he'd handcuffed my hands behind my back and had exposed my breasts and torn off my skirt.

He was standing over me, naked from the waist down, holding his large prick in his hands like some kind of arrow, his eyes greedy as they looked at my body. I tried to cover myself but he fairly fell down on me.

Funny thing, I used to think that words like cunt and prick and pussy were terrible. Now I used them like arm and leg and mouth and lips. Tits for breasts; boobs for breasts. It's sorta fun and funny to talk this way.

In any case, I don't remember everything that went on, stroke by stroke, so to speak. But I do know I screamed in terror. The more I screamed the more excited he seemed to get. Some men are like that, I guess. They like a woman to struggle; it excites them.

I wanted to vomit, but he hit me several times, then stood there, holding my face against…well, I don't like to talk about it. You can imagine what he wanted!

Some form of sanity caused me to realize that if I didn't do exactly what he said, he might kill me. I was certain he was very able to do this.

All I really know is that he raped me several times, several ways. Details. Sorry. Even if I could remember them, I…couldn't say…tell…anyway… all I know and am willing to share is that…I survived.

I did exactly what he demanded.

Well, it's easy to understand what happened. I really don't remember…I only know, logically, what happened. Obviously I blocked it all out…but I do remember that after he got his I really vomited all over him.

His reaction to that was to hit me with his fist. I remember two blows striking my face, then I lost consciousness. I never saw him again after that. I regained awareness late at night. Dazed and sick, vomiting until my stomach was convulsing on itself, I tried to tell myself it hadn't happened. But it had. I don't know how long I stayed there before gathering my torn clothes and starting for the main highway.

Several cars passed me up, one stopped, but I screamed, running away. I think this guy called the police. Because a little later a police car came along the highway and they managed to get me into their car and find out where I lived. But they took me to the hospital, and called my parents and I had to be examined and...well, all that horrible stuff. Reports made. All that. My folks didn't even come to the hospital. I never learned their reason for not coming. The police drove me home after they were finished and the doctors...well, it is somewhat of a blur. I just remember being suddenly in the house with my parents.

Dad, glared at me, he gave out a curse of anguish and fell down in a chair, unable to speak until the officers had left. I sat opposite him, hardly hearing or seeing what went on. Once the police left, Dad stood and started lecturing me, then demanding how it had happened.

Well, to be quite honest, I don't want to go into *that* part of it. I already mentioned that the folks thought I was to blame and should be cleaned of all my sins. They made me pray and do all those horrid things...every night for weeks. I hated every moment of it. I hated Dad and I hated Mom for years after that. Only in the last few years have I been able to forgive them to some extent. After all, parents aren't Gods, they are human beings and they can do some pretty terrible things. I really don't want much to do with the folks, but I can forgive and *forget*! I just like to forget all about them and what they stood for. I guess that's part of the reason for my turning away from any form of religion or God. I can't understand a God who would let something like rape take place and then have the parents of the girl blame her, in His name.

Dave has tried to make me understand something about God and Gods and religions, but I won't go for most of it. But that doesn't really matter.

I think that the main reason I managed to get over the shock of what had happened, and overcome what might have caused me to hate men for life, was my folks' attitude toward me. They considered me something like a tramp, sinful and dirty. And if you're going to have the name, you might as well have the game.

There were a lot of things that influenced me over the next years.

You know how girls will get together and talk, and sex and boys will come into the conversation. Usually there will be one or more girls who have either had a man or claim to have had one.

So you learn that sex is supposed to be fun and that there are some guys who really swing and that if you get in the right group, you can have a real "adult" time of it all. I talked with one girl—we had become pretty good friends—and she was a little on the wild side. She came from a big family that didn't have much money and she had learned a girl could get a lot of things, simply by screwing.

The thing is that she really liked to screw, and she liked to talk real dirty about it—at least, what we thought was pretty wild at that time, though now I really don't think much about such language.

She told one story that had a surprising effect on me. It was about her first experience with a couple of boys. I'll try to tell you, as best I can, to give you a pretty good idea of how I learned that sex can, after all, be fun. This made me want to try a boy my own size: for thrills!

Her story went something like this. She went to visit a boy friend, whose older brother was there. They were alone in the house, and since she had been screwing the younger brother, they got to talking about sex and they decided to do something other than talk sex. She said: "I could hardly wait; the whole idea of a double prick session seemed just the greatest. The two boys got undressed and then I followed their example. I got down on my knees before them. They stood next to each other. And I said something to them like, 'I want to eat your meat.' They dug that. So I started really having myself a double ball. Actually four balls, if you want the truth! And a couple of cocky pricks, hard as hell! I went to the older brother and fondled his balls and prick, then as it got real big, I got hold of his shaft, pointed it towards me. While I was doing this, I reached out and jerked off younger brother's red-hot cock." She told me that she just loved to eat a man, and couldn't get enough of this. "Love sucking and gulping on him. Feeling his prick belch in my mouth, jerking as I turn him on with my tongue and lips. And cumming, oh, that's just delicious. A real cocktail, if you ask me!" Afterwards she insisted that each of them service her pussy with their pricks.

The whole thing suddenly had me so hot, just listening to her, that I couldn't stand it. I asked if she knew any boys we might pick up, that I just had to have one.

The funny thing, I didn't even think about how horrible that rape had been. It was three years in the past, anyway. She knew a boy named Bob and we called him up. She said there was another girl with her who wanted to have a real sex party and that if he could find some other guy, we'd really give them a good time.

We were in her home and the boys arrived half an hour later.

Everything happened that afternoon. It was my first real experience in orgasm. There's something really voluptuously exciting about being naked in front of two men at once. This time I had the power; all of it. The idea of the four of us, naked, necking in the living room, then finally screwing, just turned me on. There's really nothing more wild than having others around while you're being screwed, or watching the others while you feel a big prick in your swollen pussy.

I've learned what a wonderful sensation it is to feel a man's hard prick in me. I just love to feel the velvet hotness of his prick and the little twitching my hips can cause to run down its long shaft.

I've had a lot of experience with men. There are things a girl can do with a man's prick. I once had three men going at once. That was sensational! Once I was eating one guy, bending over on him, while another stuck up my ass. And I was cumming. You can believe that!

I hope such admissions aren't shocking. They really shouldn't be, because sex is a physical thing that everybody feels to one degree or another.

The way I'm living right now is really the best thing in the world. For a girl like me, who just has to have pricks all over the place at once, it's just wonderful. Sometimes I dream about things like having one under each arm, one in each hand, one under each kneecap, being squeezed! One everywhere! Of course it's impossible to have anything quite that wild. But there's nothing too far out or so wild that I wouldn't embrace it with all my body. Sometimes I just want to be smothered by them! One after another.

Once, I was so overwhelmed that I started rubbing my hard tits against Dave's prick, whipping back and forth.

Another thing I just dig the most is a chain. The other night I was going down on Dave and Ralph was screwing my hot pussy, and Ann was kneeling over me in such a position that Ralph could eat her. That was wild, because Dave was going to town on Laura and Laura was blowing Jimmy. I was the only one getting a double service-job and it was just wonderful!

But that first time with the two boys was something. One of them went to work on my cunt, driving me wild. It was the first time anybody did anything like that to me. I'd never known what a pleasure that was. It so excited me that I managed to get the point across to him that I wanted to start playing with his prick. He liked that idea, so he turned, straddled my face, his balls and prick hanging between his legs just over me. He was still hot to continue, so he turned around again and shoved his prick into my sex-lips, deep, thrusting and thrusting until I had so many cums I lost count.

That's the way it is with me. I just go ape for a male! I'll eat cock any time or day. Ever since then, I just haven't been able to get enough of sex and one man would not do the job for me for very long.

I was having an affair with one guy once, but I cheated. I just couldn't stand not having something different.

That's why I dig this arrangement we have now.

Dave is just wonderful as a lover, but that's not enough for me. I have to have it down and dirty and with more than one guy at once. Well, at least much of the time!

Like, once I saw Jimmy with Ann and I just got so hot I had to help along, and we had a real swinging session.

But, I should be telling about how I got into this whole thing, I guess.

You have to understand that until I had that ball with the other couple in the living room, my first screw since being a rape—which hardly counts as a pleasant thing—I didn't really know what sex was about.

From that moment on I couldn't get enough of what men could offer. Dave told me that probably this had to do with the fact that I'd been so repressed by my folks—and had something to do with rebelling against their reaction toward me.

But hell, if you're going to be called a whore, you might as well act like one.

And I find it so fantastic playing it that way! Whoring with any hot cock that wants to sink into my body.

You have to understand that a girl who learns that sex is fun, after all, and is brought up in a family that is anti-sexual, then you really flip out.

I learned a lot after that double session, during which time I got me two male pricks. We changed boys and started all over that afternoon. It was some education, I'll tell you.

Once a girl has had sex, she wants more. And more. And more. Sometimes I go crazy just thinking about having a cock in my hands or mouth or pussy. Or all three at once. Once you've had a good one you want it again and again. That's for sure, all right. I know one girl who is frightened of sex and she said to me that it seemed that every girl that had sex wanted more and couldn't control herself, thus she was saving it. Who knows what for, because she was in her late twenties!

I feel sorry for girls who think they have to "save it" for some guy. They don't know what they are missing.

Like I said, there's nothing like a prick to give a girl joy.

For a while I ran around with a pretty wild gang of kids. We'd have sex parties, though our folks never knew what was going on. *My* folks would have guessed, simply because they thought I was sinful. Dad's attitude about the rape was that where there's fire there has to be some coals. He believed that I'd asked for it; maybe just being a woman was enough to ask for sex. I don't know what kind of sex-life he had with mother, but I can imagine. Probably went to Confession after screwing her.

Oh, I'll tell you, how I *hate* squares! They make me sick to the stomach. We've all talked about that, and the world in general, and we think people are crazy. You can have violence and killing on television, but don't have anything sexy on it. People feel it is better to read about, and see on television news reports, killing, violence, war—but they get all shaken up when something starting with S and ending with X is mentioned. Like my folks. You don't know what it does to a girl when her parents are such finks. I can't understand why Laura has such a hang-up about having seen her mother screwing. Well, enough said on *that* subject!

I certainly wouldn't want to bring kids into the world. Not this one. Not unless a lot of changes are made. I think it would be better for children to be given open sexual training and told how to protect themselves. You can't hide your head in the sand and say: they won't have sex. Because they certainly will. Maybe children should be given birth control pills—girls, that is—when they reach the age of sex. What would be wrong with that? There are too many women living off the government, because they have kids by some man who won't marry them or support the children. Instead of giving a woman money, they should give her Pills. And if she has another kid, she gets less money, *not* more! Today there's no reason for a woman getting pregnant against her wishes. Oh, there's rape, as I well know, and I was probably lucky to escape getting a kid by that bastard. I hope he's rotting in hell! But that's beside the point.

As for marriage. *That's outdated in today's world.* Unless you want kids, of course. But I think kids should be outdated, too. Well, not completely. But we have the over-population thing.

I left home when I was eighteen. I couldn't wait to get away from the folks. I'd learned a lot about sex by that time. Like I said, I'd been running around with a real swinging high school bunch. We'd have parties where couples would go off into some bedroom and screw. There was this one guy, who had a motor bike, whom I really dug. He had muscles all over him and had a real large prick between his legs. When he was dressed in jeans, you *know* how tight *they* are, you could see all his meat pressing against the crotch. I used to like putting my hand between his legs and feeling that big swelling thing. When it got real large and hard, I'd unbutton his jeans and get my face between his legs and really go to town.

Well, Harv, that was the guy's name, he wanted to split town after we'd all finished with high school. I wanted the same thing, so we took off, right after graduation. I sent a wire to the folks saying to not worry, because I was old enough to leave home and that was exactly what I had done. That was to stop the cops from searching for me. I learned later that Dad tried to get the cops on my tail, but they told him that since I was over eighteen, there really wasn't anything they could do. A girl that age has the right to leave home. I'd left, split the scene.

But it was different with Harv. His folks did get the cops on our tail. You see, he was underage, so to speak.

Anyway, we had put something like two hundred miles between us and home-town, before darkness fell. We pulled the motor bike off the road, set up camp under a real big tree and rolled out his large sleeping bag, into which both of us squeezed, naked.

It was really something being so closely pressed against a naked male body. I felt his prick going up almost immediately.

He said: "Let's screw, Nancy."

I laughed and reached for his hard prick, pushed it between my thighs and squeezed them together. Oh, I'll tell you that is something.

I certainly like to get on top of a man, get the tip of his big prick against my cunt and just move on it, not getting his meat inside mine, but just rubbing and rubbing, keeping it going like that until he can't stand it any longer, then I let the beautiful thing get inside my moist pussy and I lift up, sitting on him and the feel of his prick so large and big inside me, held captive, sends me to quick orgiastic pleasure.

With Dave you can do that kind of thing for a long time. He has wonderful control. I just keep moving my hips in slow little jerks and circles, feeling the point of his prick against my cunt, moving and teasing the flesh and nerves, all the time thinking how great it's going to be when I let him in. Then I'll slip his prick into my cunt and squeeze down hard, wanting to swallow the whole thing, shaft and all the balls between the vise of my muscles. I sometimes have the desire to squeeze it off, and keep it all for myself. I was doing that to Dave in the living room, during a sex party, one night, and some visitor with real big meat, came over, straddled his legs on each side of Dave. I had just taken Dave into my pussy and had sat up on him. Well, all at once I see this other guy facing me, his hard just in front of my mouth and I came right then at the sight.

The guy said: "Blow me, baby!"

I didn't need a second invitation. I gripped his thighs and started going to town on his hot prick while Dave began hitting me with his hips, sorta wiggling and thrusting and squirming under me. It was just great!

I know that sounds pretty terrible. But I want to be honest and tell everything about myself and the group. That's what you want, isn't it? So, I guess this is part of it. I'm only trying to point out that I just go crazy for a man!

Well, here I was in the countryside, in a sleeping bag with Harv, with his prick between my thighs. I rolled over on top of him and started moving my cunt against his prick, just feeling the end of it; moving so it was like his prick was licking my pussy. The sensations were really great. I went crazy after a very short time, getting so hot that I couldn't stand it any longer, so I managed to slide myself downwards, until I'd taken the full length of his shaft inside me. He took over then, working himself in and out faster and faster. We were making some pretty wild sounds. I had an orgasm as some flashlights hit my face.

The cops had arrived.

We were taken to the station and by morning I was back at my father's home. He started to take off his belt and I guess he was going to really beat the shit out of me. I simply ran to the front door, opened it and got out of the house as fast as possible. I'd somehow picked up my father's car keys on the stand at the front door. I ran to the car, got in and drove away. I figured Dad was the kind of bastard who would call "Cops," so I got rid of the car fast.

Here I was, without funds, hunted by the police. It was sorta exciting, now that I look back at it. The cops never found me this time, though. I remembered this wild girl I'd known in high school, the one who had taught me the real tricks—like digging sex. That one who had called up the two boys. So I went to where she was living in a run-down apartment. She was in bed with some man twice her age, both of them naked and asleep when I arrived.

Well, to make it short and sweet, she got rid of her sex partner and we lived together for a few days. She had a job at a restaurant and was able to make male contacts. I got a job at a bar, but that was a mistake, because one of Dad's friends was there, he called the folks and when Dad walked in, he made a real scene—so big that the cops were called. They put him straight—and me straight, too. It just couldn't go on like this.

That night I borrowed fifty dollars from the girl and got a bus ticket out of town.

There were a lot of towns and a lot of men before I ended up in Los Angeles. By now I was pretty expert at making the scene with men and at blocking unwanted passes in bars. I worked as a cocktail waitress most of the time, because a girl gets bigger tips and she can pick up some guy, if she wants to, and she can sleep all day. I liked the life.

You know, when I tell it this way, I wonder what kind

of life I really lived, then.

I'd get up about one or two in the afternoon, that is if I hadn't picked some prick up the night before, and then go shopping, hanging around stores, talking to strangers. I think I was terribly lonely.

By the time it was five, I'd be back at my small one bedroom apartment, fixing a canned dinner or TV dinner, watch the early show and then get ready for work. I worked until after two, then I'd either take some guy home or go home alone, have some drinks in my apartment, drinking myself to sleep.

I'll tell you, a girl can get terribly lonely living that way. People need companionship. One-night stands can give it for a moment, it's sex, so you don't have to think about loneliness.

I've talked to a lot of girls, some who lived much like I did, and they felt that having a man up at their apartment was the only thing that kept them sane. Some of the girls didn't even like sex very much. I remember one, who was going pretty steady with one man. But things were getting pretty bad. She told me something of it and I learned that she didn't like sex too much and even when she did enjoy it she was afraid to show her reactions. I flipped at that. One thing a girl learns fast, men like a woman to react. The more they react the better things will be.

Like Dave told me: *Men have great big egos and they have to have the girl show how great sex is.* How great *he* is!

That's a funny thing, Dave didn't know about me—I mean the kind of life I lived or the kind of woman I was until we started living with the group. I had to play the romantic game with him.

It's really funny, considering what I told the girl with her man troubles. I told her if she wanted to keep her fellow, she had to start putting it on strong, making him think she really dug him, prick and all. Men *love* to have their pricks worshipped, *makes them feel all man.*

When I met Dave, I was working as a secretary. I'd gotten sick and tired of the night-life and the loose passes, and the loneliness. There's something terribly lonely about working as a cocktail waitress. You're surrounded with people, but they are either with other people or are simply on the make.

So I went to school to learn what was necessary to become a secretary working. He was pretty nice. It was a long time before he approached me for a date and even then we didn't screw after dining and dancing. I tried to make it obvious what I wanted, but he didn't bite.

Well, maybe I should tell this in some detail, because then you'd understand something about Dave.

He was sensitive and very nice. I learned later that he believed there should be something between a girl and man before sex-time.

He told me some months later that it had been difficult as hell not to make a pass, because he had a hard on most of the time we were together.

I don't know what was wrong with me.

Usually when I dated a guy I would be between his legs as soon as possible.

But...well, maybe there was something about David. *I didn't want to shock him.* I liked the guy.

We danced, and I could feel his hard against my stomach and thighs and I really wanted it so bad that it hurt, but he was being so damned respectful.

He'd told me during dinner that he thought I was such a nice woman and that there were so few of them left. I asked what he meant by that and he said there were too many who were trampish. I thought, how sweet and innocent he was. His statements really flattered me.

Well, when you meet a guy who shows you respect, what can you do? I didn't want to ruin a good thing. Every girl would like to have a guy who really cares about her as a *human being*—not just a hole to shove himself in and fill up with male sperm. That's the trouble with most guys. If a girl gives herself easily to him, he thinks of her as nothing but a hole to fill. When I think of that, I shudder sometimes.

I'm not a fool, and I don't kid myself about the kind of woman I was for some time. But there were a lot of pressures shoving me in that direction. First my folks, who actually blamed me for being raped; and then a hot need for sex.

I remember the time that Dave told me about Jimmy and Laura, Ralph and Ann, who were living together, mutually sharing expenses and partners. The idea was real groovy, as far as I was concerned. And by then we'd grown to know one another fairly well; enough to be pretty honest about ourselves and sex.

We'd been living together for some time.

But I should tell you something more about Dave and myself, first.

It was some weeks before anything really happened. Oh, we kissed in the car, and his hands found my breasts. It drove me crazy. I really wanted to go all the way, but felt it would be a mistake to make the first move.

Finally he did come out and say: "Honey, you're really getting to me!" That was after some hot session in his car, outside of my apartment. "I don't know what to do about you!" he laughed, giving my body a real look, like he wanted to go all the way.

I did what any realistic girl in my position might do. He wanted to make love to me; I wanted the same thing, and either one of us came out and stated it, or we'd go nuts—or something like that.

So I said: "Dave, I don't see anything wrong with a man and woman who care about one another, building a real relationship. It's driving me crazy, too!"

He laughed at that, pulled me into his arms, and we

kissed real passionately. Without any more words, the two of us went up to my apartment. He carried me into the bedroom and started making love to me like no man had ever done before.

Usually, when you start sexing it with a guy, you get undressed and bang away. There's no build up, nothing but mutual orgasm desired and received. Wild clawing and ravishing one another.

But Dave lay me on the bed and slowly caressed my clothes off, piece by piece. Those touches drove me wild and I just couldn't wait for him to get undressed. He'd been doing things like touching my thighs, running his hand across my pussy and then up to my breasts as he pulled blouse and then bra off. I was real hot, all over.

And the way he talked. It was wonderful. Things like telling me how beautiful my legs and breasts were. He would expose some portion of my body, say how lovely it was, how crazy he was about me, then start caressing and kissing my flesh until it was burning. He was damned good at it, too. But by the time I was naked, I just couldn't wait, so I grabbed at him, drawing his body down against mine, pressing my swollen cunt against his crotch where I could feel a real long and large prick under his slacks. Oh, that just drove me wild and I slipped my fingers between us, fumbled until I'd managed to unzip his pants. He helped then, until we had his hard cock exposed. I put it between my thighs and we embraced, tongue kissing. His hands cupped my breasts, then he started kissing their hard nipples, going from one to the other. All the time my thighs kept squeezing on his prick, moving as best I could so I could feel it slipping and squirming between my legs. It drove me out of my mind. Finally I just couldn't stand it any longer and somehow managed to spread my legs real wide. Then the delightful feel of his prick against my moist pussy was too much. I just drove myself up against his shaft, taking the full extent of it.

That was a crazy wonderful feeling and I just went out of my head. It was like that for weeks afterwards. We just couldn't get enough of one another. Naturally we talked about sex and what our experience before meeting each other had been. I finally told him about the rape and he almost cried for me. I've never seen such emotion. I guess I fell in love then. But it was the kind of love a woman feels when discovering that there is somebody in the world that really cares about her. This was the first time I felt important to another human being.

We started living together after a while. And when you start doing something like that, the subject of sexual freedom comes pretty quickly into your conversation. I really don't know how it all came up, but we finally admitted to each other that there really wasn't anything wrong with having sexual orgasm with other people, because it was merely physical release.

I remember Dave saying: "I've known a lot of girls, but there's a complete difference between somebody you care about and somebody you are just screwing for orgasm." He meant that I was important, better and more satisfying *because he cared about me.*

David is a romantic. He was convinced he loved me in a spiritual way; yet he kept being bothered by the fact that he could enjoy the idea of screwing somebody else. In other words, he could look at another girl and have a physical reaction. We talked about that, too. David is a big talker, I'll tell you. A brain, but all doubletalk, if you ask me. He gets so involved in his complex thoughts that there isn't any room for a more simple line of thinking.

To me it is really very simple: sex is fun; and if it is fun with one person, why shouldn't it be *more* fun with more people?

I finally told David that I didn't see anything wrong with desiring other people. I then said:

"To be truthful, there are other men I could sleep with;

but it wouldn't be as nice as with you; only different."

Well, to make a long story short, as they say, we had come to the conclusion that sexual freedom was a good thing and couldn't harm the way we felt about one another. It was that simple.

So when he came home one night, saying he'd been talking to Jimmy, at lunch, and that there was a chance we could move in with him, Laura and Ralph and Ann, all of whom we knew casually, I couldn't help thinking the idea was pretty good.

You see, we all live in a very beautiful, expensive home; none of us could afford this alone. Another thing is that nobody in the surrounding homes can guess what is going on. To them it looks like we're just three couples sharing expenses, having our own private living quarters while sharing kitchen, dining and living rooms. We hardly advertise our real attitudes to people who don't share them already. That's why we had known Ralph, Jimmy, Laura, and Ann.

Well, in any case, David and I agreed it might be a very good thing and we started to get together with the others; after a few months it was decided we all were pretty good for each other.

I guess it all could sound pretty cold, cut and dried, the way I just explained it. But you have to understand that David and I had gotten to the point where we either got married or faced the fact that continuing on the way we were going to get either of us any place. For myself, well, I really didn't want to get married. And to be truthful, it was the longest time I'd ever been with one man. I wanted a more broad sexual experience. I guess David was a little intrigued about having something more orgiastic. We had both agreed that orgies might be fun. Things like more than one couple in the same room.

We went to a small party that Jimmy and Ralph were giving. There were a few other couples, all willing to swing a little sex.

The way we played it the first party was pretty simple, really. After drinks, there were a few films. Things men see at stag parties. The full sexual thing. It really knocked me out. I'd heard about such films but never had seen one. They really go all the way. And they get the camera in a beautiful location to see men's pricks screwing cunts, real close-up. What jazzed me was seeing this woman blowing a man. She kept running her tongue along his cock, which was real large and hard, then she put her lips around the end and slowly moved them down, taking in more and more of his prick. It so excited me that I couldn't control myself. I just had to feel a prick in my hand. I reached out and started fondling one I thought to be David, but it turned out to be Ralph, and he has a real big gun. When I realized it wasn't David, I felt a real voluptuous thrill and Ralph didn't do anything to stop me. So I just unzipped his fly and started playing with him. Finally, during the end of the film, I was jerking my hand up and down on his large prick and he went off. It felt good working my fingers all over his twitching cock. I got a real charge out of it. He was re-zipping his pants when the lights went on. I saw Laura with David in the far corner of the room, her hand on his crotch, his hands fondling her breasts and crotch. They were French kissing like wild. I turned to Ralph and said: "Let's do something really good."

But instead, Jimmy suddenly stood and said:

"We're all adults and we all know what we want. Why don't we just get naked, turn out the lights and do it right."

Everybody was *hot* to sex it up and I quickly stood and slipped out of my dress pulled off my sweater and undid my bra all the time looking directly into Ralph's eyes. He's a real hairy man, large, barrel-chested, and so animal. Well, he turned me *on in a real hot sexual way.*

He got undressed, then we came into each other's arms as the lights went out. I had noticed that neither David nor

Laura had stopped making love, though they had progressed pretty far by then. David had her skirt high up and her panties down, his fingers were running along her stomach and pussy and thighs while they continued to French each other's mouths. She had been fondling and rubbing his crotch and I saw her fingers begin to work on the zipper just before the lights went out. The whole scene excited me.

Then I felt Ralph's large prick between my thighs and I started squirming and jerking my hips so I was giving his shaft a real working over with my legs. I could feel its rigid shape under my crotch and it was stimulating as hell. We frenched each other while his hands played with my butt and breast. I just couldn't wait. When he was hard enough, I shifted, lifted up high on my tip toes until the point of his prick was right at the entrance to my hot cunt. Then I surged down real slowly and thrilled to excitement as his huge meat shoved deep into mine. We fairly danced against one another. It was the first time I'd ever done it standing.

But I'll tell you one thing I've done it with Ralph like that many times since then even in the shower little more relaxed, and had a round of drinks.

Ralph suggested that we play Blind Man's Make, as he calls it.

All the girls and men are blindfolded and then they stand in the middle of the room. The whole idea is to start feeling with your hands and try to name the person you touch. The funny thing is when a man and man touch or a woman touches you. It is a strange sensation, because at first you can't tell for sure what sex is touching you. Here is where you get really sexually stimulated. Fingers reach out and touch, and suddenly you find it's a girl. Then the next set of fingers might get to your breasts and it's a man. Then you feel some hand slipping between your thighs, it fingers your pussy. Or a fanny touches your fanny. The contacts in the total blindness are exciting and continual.

The whole idea is to stand there, in a close group, reaching out, touching, searching and then fondling. I got hold of two pricks in the darkness and then felt a hand slipped between my legs, searching with trembling fingers where it was hot. Then somebody's ass touched mine and I felt another hand cup my breast and suddenly somebody managed to find my lips and we Frenched like wild. I jerked off one prick and then pulled the other low, between my legs. The two of us trembled together and slid down onto the floor and the guy really went down right between my legs, hitting my target with such beautiful skill that I gasped out in delight. Later I learned it was Jimmy.

He's real good at hitting right on target. We kept doing it for a long time. He had great control. He just kept that damned long prick of his going in and out time and time again, driving me crazy. I twisted my hips, squeezed down on it, churned up against him, did everything I could to make him cum, but he just continued the same controlled rhythm that built such pleasure that I had orgasm after orgasm, each bigger and greater than the last. When he finally strained for his climax, I went just about insane and afterwards lost consciousness for a short time.

The thing is: we really dug the scene after that party. The second party and we were convinced it would be a good idea to join up with them. We all enjoyed each other's company—which was important. And the second party was just the three couples, a try-out for a weekend. Us girls get along pretty good, too, which is important.

It's the orgy things that I lock onto. I really like having a couple of men doing me at once. That's the best. Every chance I get, I try to get at least two of the boys to come on strong with me. I dig having one screw my pussy, while I go down on another. Then it's great fun to get my hands on another prick and fondle and jerk on it. All my senses are alive to the male cock. I'm feeling one in my pussy, like a girl is supposed to, and I'm feeling one in my hands, like a girl should enjoy holding.

But, I must admit that I like these crazy games we play in the darkness, because you can't tell who is touching you. Some people don't like it because they get all bothered about being excited by a caress that comes from somebody of their own sex—I'm not talking about the group that lives in the House, they're not hung-up so much like that...other than Ann, maybe. She doesn't like it if some woman gets fresh in the darkness. But there are a lot of people who are frightened of being homosexual—you know, they think that if they get a thrill in the darkness when someone of their own sex touches them, it means they might like to have homosexual relations, and that frightens them. Scares them shitless.

I don't mind who touches me in the dark. A touch is a touch, and it's surprising how difficult it is to tell what the sex is behind the touch. If a fanny presses yours, how can you tell for sure if it's a woman or a man? It doesn't really bother me. If I get a charge out of a touch, and it happens to be a woman, what difference does it make? I know what I like. I just dig pricks and balls and can't get enough of them. *I* know I'm normal; regardless of the fact that I was raped by some damned bastard prick it didn't turn me against them.

I guess I'm just sexy.

As for my reasons for liking to live this way? Well, I would have to simply say that *it is certainly more realistic and practical.* I don't want just marriage; I want orgiastic pleasure in large lumps. I want to live while I can. You just don't know what the future is going to bring. I guess if I had been living at another time, maybe when there was an all-out war, I'd have been one of those girls who gave herself to all the boys going off to the front to get themselves killed. Give them a thrill before they die. Maybe that's what we're all doing, in a way; getting a thrill before we die.

David has said that sex is just a very important part of living and life and it took him a long time to realize it. He told me that Laura was partly responsible for this change in his attitude. But I think it was me, too—or at least *could* have been me. Not that I'm trying to prove anything. Just that I met David and liked him and wanted him to like me. I guess I wanted respectability; which I didn't really have for a long time. I admit that, now, because I don't feel any guilts about it. I understand myself. I know I like orgasm and I like male pricks. I just love to fondle them, make them get real large under my caresses or kisses, if you like. The more the better. It's fun feeling the difference. It's fun seeing how much control you have over a man's prick; how you can really get him high and then really go to town on him. I enjoy the total control a woman has over a man's prick. I know all the triggers and can decide when he's gonna cream my fingers, and not until I want him to mess me up with his delicious cum.

For me, a girl who would like to be accepted and loved and respected, but who needs more than one man as a plaything, this is the only way to live. We are just one happy, happy family. In a way, I guess, that's the nice thing about our lives. A family that cares about one another, who needs one another and accepts one another as sexual beings. There isn't any guilts or anti-sexual attitudes among us; and that's important to me. I don't want anything to do it with people who turn their noses up at sex. I want to live, exist on the fullness of sexual expression—which is the way people should be.

Not like my folks. Not like the fag civilization we live in. Really, I mean it just that way. Our society is nothing better than a Fag world. They're so anti-sexual that it's disgusting.

My childhood was filled with that anti-sexual attitude,

that horrid religious hate for life itself! My parents were monsters! They turned me off of any religious stuff for so many years. Only in the last few years have I come to terms with that...but a totally different kind of religious experience, one which embraces love in all its wonderful levels. Sharing space and pleasure like one would share a delicious meal; we just don't stop at food. We feed each other in every possible way, and it is a lovely, wonderful thing of mutual living, openly and without restrictions other than that we all want to share the same thing, together, as a group! It is simply wonderful!

And as far as love goes, well, if it's like what the folks had, I don't want any part of it. I simply want this modern, realistic life we experience. A unit, a small, simple society where people care enough about those around them to give of themselves completely.

To love one another in total, and as a sexual being.

Let's not war, let's love, screw each other in the best meaning of the word.

COMMENTS

Nancy would seem on the surface, if one was to take her words as total truth, *a very sexually centered woman,* who has a great passion and need and love for men. But in order to accept her statements as total honesty, one would have to ignore her rape experience; one would have to forget that nobody can go through such an experience without some scars; one would have to forget that her parents taught her sex was dirty, sinful, wrong.

Anybody brought up in such a social environment could hardly develop into the type of person as Nancy pictures herself to others and to herself.

There is no doubt that she is convinced that her love for men and "pricks" is normal and natural. Yet there were many indications that she is far from healthy in her outlook towards sex and love. Her childhood experience left its lasting scars, which, at least, she is dealing with as best she can; and managing to enjoy this life she had chosen for herself.

The one thing I discovered about her, she does not think of love and sex as being a united function or that it is even necessary, or necessarily desirable, to have a real love relationship. It was orgasm. A man is a prick and a woman is a hole to be filled up for the mutual need of orgasm. That, alone, is not wrong; it is only wrong when this is the *only* and final reason for sexual expression. Sex is more than just physical interaction; it involves the emotion and a lot of other things, far more basic and far more important than mere orgasm.

I saw many indications of penis-hatred in Nancy's statements. Her over-importance on the male penis, her desire to control and to devour it certainly suggested a deep-seated hatred for men and their sexual parts. And certainly understandable considering her father. Her statements about orgies in the darkness, where it was impossible to tell the difference between a male or female touch, suggested a latent homosexual desire. And while this is not a horrid thing in itself, it is a part of her experience which she is, no doubt, in denial. Is that wrong? Probably not. She's doing the best she can with what she has, and is, to some extent enjoying life. Can all of us truly claim to have done better? Adjusting to what life offers and making the most of it with whatever tools we have is certainly not such a bad thing.

She's, at least, found a way to deal. And if it is illusion, so what?

It is my belief that Nancy is doing exactly what her parents regarded as sinful and immoral, as a rebellion to their reaction to a very shocking and horrible experience: rape.

A case might be developed for her being a highly sexual woman, who was damaged early in life.

My feeling, in hearing her story, was that because of early experience, or because of the general situation of the world in general, she found the sexual-love relationship between one man and one woman, difficult to live with. She rejects the old concept of love and rationalizes into believing that sex, for sex itself and nothing more, is the real desirable state between man and woman and that love does not have to enter into it.

Perhaps she somehow relates that kind of emotional value with whatever she images her parents must have shared.

Nancy came close to a real love affair with David, but I believe because of her actual hatred of men—on a subconscious level—made it impossible to want such love, and at the same time need other men to possess and conquer.

She, more than anybody else, actually came on strong in the department of considering the group as "family."

Actually I would have liked to have done a fuller study of Nancy, probing deeper into her motives and desires, but it was impossible. I tried to question her on homosexual desires, but she simply laughed it off, saying that she'd no more desire another woman than she would desire screwing her father. An *interesting* statement in that I asked her: "Tell me, Nancy, do you ever remember thinking of your father as a sexual symbol? It's quite natural, you know, for boys to, at one time or another, desire their mother in at least a subconscious way and for girls to feel the same thing for their fathers. After all these are their most intimate role models at that maturing point of their childhood."

"Are you kidding?" she cried, much too alarmed. Then her laugh was a little loud, tense. "I sometimes think he didn't have a sexual bone in his body. Though, of course he must have. Unless I *wasn't* his daughter. Interesting thought, isn't it? He certainly didn't act like my father, *after* I was raped! I really don't want to talk about him!"

Her rejection of her father here seemed to me to indicate almost the opposite. Her reaction was *too* violent. I couldn't help feeling that she was reacting to the opposite point, rebelling to some subconscious desire that she consciously rejected. A father who had rejected her on some very basic levels.

In other words: I believe that Nancy, like any normal girl, had gotten to the state where she really felt close to her father. Then she was raped. He turned against her, rejected her when she needed him the most. What probably made it even more difficult was the fact that this was surrounded by a sexual assault; thus: *sexual* rejection! Such sexual rejection can cause a person to seek acceptance; but in an unhealthy way.

She is, in effect, accepted in this group; but doesn't go outside it, now that she found a perfect center for a certain amount of freedom.

All is speculation on my part, built on the facts presented above, in her own words. There weren't enough facts to give a total picture; but enough to cause one to desire more. She wouldn't give them.

The simple fact is: because of the kind of person she is, and the past experiences in her life, plural sex fashioned by living with other couples and sharing their lives in a total sexual way, gives Nancy the fulfillment she needs. Under different circumstances, she would unquestionably be giving herself to many men, picking them up for one night stands or for prolonged affairs and be very unhappy and lonely. She needs companionship, she needs a form of love which means acceptance. But on some basic level is in conflict with the very idea of that kind of love, not trusting it. And that's because of her father.

Under different circumstances she might have become a prostitute or turned into a sadist or Lesbian—but the curve of her life directed her to orgy sex. Circumstances brought her to a group of people that could live together, love sexually together, and accept one another on that level.

I don't believe there was anybody, other than Ralph and Ann, who desired real marital love. But their situation, as detailed in the next part of this series, turned them away from such marital bliss in a desperate search for something totally different. They were, to me, *the most tragic of the group,* because they had tried to find a normal union of man and wife and failed for reasons really beyond their control. Yet, they, too, found an answer for their cravings and frustrations in communal living.

CHAPTER FOUR

RALPH

[Author's note: this is the last of the PLURAL SEX series. And to get the full impact it is suggested that the previous three parts be read first—even though this one is, as the others, complete in itself. The four, together, build a more complete picture that gives their arguments for couples living together, sharing their lives in an intimate union of plural sex. My conclusions at the end of this case-history cover some of the other couple's views.]

Ralph is a big, muscular man with sandy hair and a ruddy, rugged face. But, while there is humor in his eyes, there is also a deep sense of pain. He and his wife, Ann, tried marriage and have kept to it. They love one another, yet have found great pain in this love. It is best to let Ralph tell his story, without any more statements about him or his marriage or Ann.

* * * * * * *

I can remember many things in my childhood that were of a sexual nature. I masturbated all throughout my teens, even after having had my first girl. I had a very deep need for sexual expression right from the beginning. There weren't any restrictions of this nature put upon me; but there wasn't any attention given either one way or the other by Mother.

My folks had divorced early, when I was about four. I really don't remember much about living with both of them. There is a vague memory of having both in the same house, hearing screaming voices. They fought a lot.

Mother, I think, was a virgin when she married Dad. My father either found her unfulfilling as a sexual partner or emotionally unrewarding. I really don't know for sure.

I do know what they both told me over the years. Mother claimed that Dad didn't have any consideration for her as a woman, and that he cheated fairly early in their married life. Dad claimed that Mother was sexually cold to his advances. I also learned that Mother couldn't have any children after I was born. Dad wanted a big family. He finally remarried and had several children with his second wife before she was killed in an auto accident. After that he simply played the field until he reached the age of fifty, when he married his secretary for companionship.

Mother, as far as I can reason it out, lived a secluded life for a few years after the divorce, though I believe she did have a couple of affairs immediately after the divorce. Then later, when I was about ten or eleven, she started dating a lot of men, most of which would usually end up spending the night with her. This went on until I was fifteen, when she married a man about six years younger than she was.

By then I was too interested in girls to be bothered with my home-life, which swung between Mother and Dad. I usually wanted to stay with Dad, because they had such a nice home life, until his second wife was killed. Her name was Helen and I think I probably had a crush on her when I was in my early teens. Maybe that was natural, maybe not.

At some point, I suppose, I probably should have had a

crush on my mother; that relationship was a strange one. She didn't resent me; but actually flooded me with a lot of love.

I guess I was almost smother-loved by her. Considering I was her only child. She told me that the most important thing a person can have is children; their own.

Helen, my father's wife, really turned me on one day, when I was visiting them. She was a woman with a beautiful body, wide hips and full breasts, long black hair that fell to her shoulders. She was sun-bathing at their pool, had on a two-piece swim suit. I just couldn't get my eyes off her. She must have noticed my interest in her body, because she said: "You're getting interested in girls, aren't you?"

But it was not meant to be a sexual remark. She would never have thought of even suggesting anything between the two of us; though I might have submitted to seduction if that had been what she wanted.

I admitted to being interested and she said that it was healthy for a boy my age to like girls. "Just remember that girls are much like boys, Ralph. Just be nice to them. Don't take advantage of their innocence."

She was sitting up, starting to stand for a dive in the pool, when her bathing suit top fell slightly and I saw a rounded white breast and the pink tip of a nipple.

That night I really went to town on my dick, working it up and down, thinking about Helen and that naked breast. I knew enough to know men liked to kiss and suck women's breasts—and I certainly wanted to put that nipple of hers into my mouth.

She had covered herself without comment, but I'm quite sure she'd seen the look of immediate lust in my eyes. A couple of days later Dad got me aside and told me the basic facts of life. I believe that Helen had talked to him and suggested this. It was really quite pointed and he didn't seem at all embarrassed. He told me just about everything a boy should know. Once he'd established I knew about sex, he went about telling me how to protect a woman and then told me things about how a woman is, what she desires and how to satisfy her. When he told about cunnilingus, the whole idea seemed crazy, but it fascinated me. When he said that some women liked to perform fellatio on a man, I found that even more exciting. in fact the whole conversation excited me so much that I couldn't wait to get a woman and discover what it might be like.

Dad told me that the first girl he'd had was a woman about ten years older than himself and that he'd been lucky to have the experience, because she told him a lot about sex. "I was just about your age at the time, son," he said. "It was really a very nice experience."

Somehow I managed to say that he had been lucky and I only wished it could happen to me that way. I really don't know how I managed to tell him that, because I was terribly embarrassed. Maybe that was part of the reason I did say it; trying to show how sophisticated I was; *hide* my embarrassment. Probably he saw through that, too. But he did say he knew a woman who was very highly sexed and he thought it would be possible to arrange something. I learned later that she was a prostitute, though one who charged a big bill for her services. Well, a call-girl, really. And, most important was the fact that she actually did like sex. There aren't many such women. But Dad was in a business which used the services of call-girls to put across deals and he knew quite a few professionals in the field. He told me some years later that he'd gone to a call-girl he knew, told her the situation and asked if she knew any girl who really liked sex, one that could teach his son what it was like with a real woman.

It turned out she knew one girl in her middle twenties who had gone into the profession on a part-time basis, to get extra money and because she really couldn't get enough sex.

I'll call her Gina, because she was Latin, with lovely wide hips, a flat stomach, dark smoldering eyes, a generous mouth and full, bouncy breasts. And I mean that her breasts were really bouncy.

Dad told me about the set-up, though not that she was a professional or that he had paid a hundred dollars for her to teach me about sex. He offered to take me there and I accepted this arrangement. He stayed long enough to make introductions.

Gina was wearing a fluffy robe, which showed little other than the fact that she didn't have anything on underneath. Once Dad had left, she smiled at me and asked if I had ever seen a naked woman. I shook my head, and she simply opened her robe, let it fall to the floor.

She had such a magnificent body, like some Goddess. Her breasts were full, rounded, their nipples high, pert, cherry pink. Her waist dipped in and then beautiful hips, real plush, circled out down to fully developed, lovely tapering thighs and legs. I do believe she was just about the most beautiful woman I ever saw; almost too beautiful.

I looked at her breasts like I couldn't get enough of looking, then at her stomach, which was flat, but fleshy in a nice sensual way, the navel tucking in like some little dot. Her pubic area was already swelled slightly. I think just being naked like that, before a young boy, who is totally innocent of sexual knowledge, excited her very much.

I wanted to touch her so very much that when she stepped forward in a swivel-hipped fashion I found it very easy—in fact impossible to do anything else!—to reach out. My hands fell naturally to her hips.

That's something I should say, I guess, right now. I find it very exciting to have my hands on a woman's hips. I like the feel of them, soft and round, firm. During intercourse, I'll many times grip a woman's hips, if it's possible, and move them up and down to match my strokes. I guess it's some kind of fetish with me. I just can't get enough of holding a woman's hips, moving them; or just being aware of their own movement, if the girl knows what to do.

I was really quite hard by that time. The moment my hands touched the softness of her hips. Her flesh was very hot.

She immediately started to undo my belt and pants, saying: "Here, let me help you. We both want to be naked, you know. I just love seeing a man's... penis." In a little while she didn't use such nice terms. I know now that she wanted to say the more blunt word, but had hesitated when realizing it might shock me.

Her hands pulled the pants down around my hips, then I felt her fingers touch my erection where it pressed against my underpants.

"You are very large for a young man your age!" She admired me in a pleased voice. Then slowly she worked my underpants down so that I was fully exposed and her fingers searched my shaft, working from the tip down along the full length until she found my balls, which she squeezed lightly, gently, and thrillingly. Damned she made that really good!

Instinct and what Dad had told me about sex, caused me to pull her hips against mine and the feel of her pubic hair against my shaft and balls was overwhelming. I was dazed and dizzy from that moment on. Slowly her fingers were working my pants lower and lower; then she started sliding down, bending, so it was possible to get the pants about my ankles. She helped me step out of them, then sat up so that her face was directly in front of my prick.

"You are very large and manly," she observed, eyes glistening. She moistened her lips with a pointed pink tongue.

I then said something pretty funny, in a way, now that

I think of it. But it was logical and the right thing to say. I asked: "Are you going to kiss it?" I was so fascinated by what Dad had told me about fellatio that I really wanted her to do that.

She smiled, ran her tongue along her full lips, looked up at me and asked: "You want me to?"

I managed a nod.

"Oh, that's delightful!" she exclaimed in a high pitched, happy voice. "I wanted to, but wasn't sure if you might not be shocked."

Trying to sound very mature and bold, I said:

"Well, Dad told me all about sex, and I liked everything he told me. I want to kiss yours, too, if you'll let me."

"Delightful!" she exclaimed again. But this time her lips were very close to my hard and I could feel the breath of her words against it.

Then her tongue slipped out between her moist lips and touched lightly at the base of my shaft and worked its way up flicking slightly back and forth until it reached the crown, where it twirled around and around while her lips slipped slowly about the tip. When she started pulling it into her mouth I began twitching from excitement and she guessed I'd burst in moments. After all, nothing like this had ever been done to me, and nobody can take that kind of punishment for long—first time around. So she pressed her soft lips real hard on the shaft and pushed her tongue up against the bottom of the head and tugged on my penis real hard, her tongue moving back and forth. The stimulation was far too great and I just went off like an explosion. By then her lips had released me and as I recovered, she took my hand and led me across the room to a long, low couch where we lay down together, her thighs against mine, side by side, arms about one another.

I was aware of the softness of her breasts and the hard points of her nipples.

She held me that way for some time, then her thighs opened and her hand took hold of my limp, retarded penis, pulled it out and clamped her warm thighs about it. The feel was erotic, but it was going to take a few minutes before I would be able to really start reacting to this intimate sexual contact.

She reached around behind me and put her fingers between my legs, caressing and teasing my balls, all the time her lips started kissing mine and we Frenched. I found my own hand automatically searching for her breast, and when I found one ripe nipple, I caressed it lovingly.

It didn't take long before I was really high and hurting and she didn't wait to give me a chance to do the real thing to her. Once she felt my hard had developed size and shape, she rolled over on her back, pulling me with her, then with her fingers, she pointed my prick right at the entrance to her moist hot cunt and started to urge it inside. I didn't need more than that to get the idea. I thrust down with all my weight. She moaned slightly, then grinning up at me, said:

"Lift your weight up with your hands and arms, like you were doing push-ups. Ride me gently."

I must admit that this first one was pretty good. Somehow I managed to keep up for about ten or so strokes and each one was more heavenly. Of course, she had ways to keep me going. Her legs clamped tightly about mine and her hips kept moving so it was impossible to escape her; and she clamped down hard on my prick so it was held securely inside her moist sexual cavity. Another point had helped; her going down on me like she had. I guess that's why she went to it so passionately and directly; to get the first orgasm out; to lower the lusting pressure.

Afterwards she went into the bathroom and washed herself real good. She told me, when returning, that she was squeaky clean, then came down and lowered her head on my prick.

"Want to suck mine?" she inquired.

I readily found that very exciting, so she straddled my face, lowering her crotch down to my lips. It was a fascinating sight. Then she started slowly to go to work on my penis with tongue and lips, gently, carefully, making certain that I got the idea that this was supposed to last a long time. She said a few things, in-between voluptuous kisses. Things like, "Run your tongue gently between my lips, there. Kiss me like you would kiss my mouth. Do it gently, like I'm doing to you."

I got the idea.

It was something doing a sixty-nine with her. She took her time on me and didn't force me to start until I was ready. I lay there, bathed in the sensations of her kisses, looking up at the heart shape of her crotch, getting more and more excited. Then I placed my hands on her hips and found myself planting a gentle kiss on her pussy. She responded by pulling more voluptuously on my hard with her soft lips.

I guess the reason I'm telling about this in such detail is because it impressed me. This was my first experience with a woman and I was finding every activity very exciting. I've heard about other men's first experiences in doing these variations on the sex act and they admit to being revolted, while at the same time unable to control their urges to do them. I found them delightful. I just was swimming in joy at what was happening.

That first pussy kiss and her responding action drove me to hotter and hotter kisses until we were really going to hell and back on one another.

Man, I'll tell you one thing, to me there's nothing like doing this kind of thing with a woman!

And she couldn't get enough of it; believe me. She just couldn't get enough.

After we'd finished with that, she continued to mouth my penis, but changed positions so that her face was facing mine, from behind my legs. After a while she sat up, straddled my hips and started using her cunt on my penis, which was getting a little excited by then. She was expert and excited enough to make a fag get hard. She took her time, doing things like leaning over me and brushing her large tits against my chest, moving back and forth, while her pussy, down on the end of my shaft, circled over the tip, up and down, back and forth. When I was about to burst with the excitement of what was doing, her body lifted upwards and then surged down, engulfing my shaft with the moist walls of her swollen hot sex-cave. We rammed together time and again until orgasm blew both our heads off.

Neither of us could go another round after that. We lay in bed, sleeping, for half the night. But I was awakened by her hands fondling me and her lips covering mine. We did another round then, in darkness. This time she left me totally spent out, doing just about everything we'd done before, but never to orgasm until we'd entered sexual coupling. But this time the position was different. She got on her knees, bent over, so her fanny was high up, thighs spread, and told me to enter her from that position. It was really something feeling her fanny cheeks against my hips as I entered her vagina. I hammered away after that for a long time.

I've discovered it is really great to do this kind of thing, entering either a woman's cunt or her ass. You can grip her hips and then ram yourself again and again at her, harder and harder, almost brutally. There's something savagely exciting about this kind of position.

Afterwards we fell asleep again and the next morning I left, a total man in my carnal knowledge of women. The kind of woman I have always demanded since.

A couldn't wait to get a girl my own age. But Dad had pointed out one thing, which I have gone by since then: don't go out trying to seduce a virgin.

I've had virgins, but it was merely by accident. There was only one other woman like Gina, before I married Ann. In this I mean that Ann is really great in bed; one of the best sex-partners a man might have as a wife. And I guess that sounds strange, considering that I like to have it with other women. But I'll go into that a little later, because it's important.

I had a lot of girls during high school. There were some who would only let me finger their pussy, because they were frightened of a man's prick. Others would go down on me, but wouldn't let me pop their cherry, which they were saving for their future husbands.

I've always respected a girl's wishes.

In any case, I was working in a hotel for a while, during summer, and there was this other woman, working in the cocktail lounge, who really lived a pretty wild life. There was a room in the back of the clerk's desk for the night man. That was me. You didn't have to be out front all the time.

Well, this girl, call her Terry, came in late from the cocktail lounge, after work, drunk as hell. She asked if she could use the boy's room for the night-clerk's sleeping quarters. I let her. She went in and then came out a little later, dress half off, bra removed.

She looked at where I was lying on the bed reading—there was a buzzer that would tell me if anything was needed in the lobby—and said, "Can I lay down there, honey?"

I looked at her body and got a quick reaction. Her dress was half open at the top, and it was obvious she was naked under it.

I nodded and she lay down real close to me, tapped the book I was reading and asked: "Is it sexy?"

I shook my head. "Not really."

"I like sexy books, don't you?" she inquired, looking up into my eyes like a wanton bitch in heat.

"I don't like to read about sex," I told her quite honestly.

"What's wrong, don't you like girls?"

"Too much to only read about them."

She laughed at that, then asked: "How much do you like girls?"

I stared at her, closed the book, then said:

"Enough to know what to do when one is attractive to me."

"Am attractive to you?" she inquired, running a finger along my lips.

For answer I simply reached out and put my hand under her dress, against the naked flesh of her breast.

She squirmed against my hand and said:

"That's more like it. I want a piece real bad."

Immediately we were at it. There was a chance that somebody might come into the lobby, so I felt a frantic need to be done with it. She felt the same need for speed, and quickly reached down and got my penis out, fondling it. I lifted up her skirt and she was naked there, too. But the sight of that naked pussy drove me to a fit. Her hips were wide, her thighs real meaty and I couldn't help myself. I covered her thighs, stomach and finally her pussy with hot kisses. She lay back, moaning and squirming in orgiastic pleasure.

By the time she had had several spasms that could have been orgiastic climaxes, I couldn't take any more of it and so I thrust my erected penis deep into her hot cunt and hammered away. She had several other climaxes before I'd blown my head.

But it was far from over. I was about to redress when she sat up, grabbed my hips and started covering my crotch with hot voluptuously passionate tongue kisses. Somehow she managed to tell me to finger her, so I put my hand against her pussy and did just that.

It wasn't over even then. She wanted it every way,

again and again. Luckily we weren't interrupted once during the night and we continued on a sexual orgy that would have knocked most people dead.

The thing I'm trying to put across is that I need a voluptuously passionate woman; I need orgasm more than most men. All during my pre-marital relations I seldom found it necessary to use a rubber. Usually the girl claimed to need it real badly and said she could take care of herself.

No girl got pregnant because of intercourse with me. Maybe that should have warned me.

It didn't.

When I met Ann, we dated, fell madly in love, but didn't have sexual intercourse before marriage. Ann wanted to be a virgin for the man she married. I respected this. But we did do other things. We did mutual masturbation, and I taught her the pleasure of anal intercourse after we'd become engaged. We both wanted children. That was very important and she said this once:

"I never want to wear anything that might stop pregnancy or have you do so, or use any birth-control measure—not until we have the right number of children. And I don't want to have a child out of wedlock." That ended all thought of this kind of screwing before marriage.

On the wedding night we got naked and she made love to my penis like she had never done before; but not to orgasm. She caressed and caressed my shaft and balls with loving fingers, used her lips and tongue to keep it erect while I serviced her vagina with my lips. It was agreed without any words, to make the first time last as long as possible, but to make the first orgasm and all those that followed, to flood deep within her body. "I don't want to throw away any of that precious liquid," she had told me. "It might be a child—our *first* child."

I held off and then we came into each other's arms, hips pressed gently together. I rolled her over on her back

124

and then slowly, carefully inserted my penis into the entrance to her vagina.

Knowing the first thrust would probably hurt her, I tried to make it swift and yet at the same time as gentle as possible. I positioned myself so that this first penetration would go in straight, sliding down the channel of her vagina in such a way that it couldn't hurt her any more than possible.

She moaned, both in pain and in a release of pleasure, as she later told me. I let my penis rest deep within her for a long time as we savored this first wonderful sensation of our union. I have never experienced anything like that moment; before or afterwards. This was the woman I loved and the first penetration into her very soul.

But on the second stroke, Ann moaned, "Oh, you're wonderful!"

I'd never known such a beautiful feeling as when she said those words. It was the first time I had entered a woman I loved; and that alone made it completely different from any other female body I'd possessed. Each stroke was timed with loving care, each penetration made it more beautiful and thrilling. I kept thinking things like:

This is the woman I love and we are making love together to have a child. There's something beautiful about that; something wonderful.

Afterwards, Ann embraced me and we lay in each other's arms for a long time, then she started fondling my penis and told me to just lay there while she loved me, worshipped my manhood. But she didn't want to waste the seed of life and before I could go off, she thrust herself upon my shaft, gulping upon the spray of my explosion. For we wanted to have children right away.

The next day and night we made love time and time again, usually filling her vagina with what we hoped would be a future child. We had timed our marriage and honeymoon so that it was between her periods—spreading out over the two weeks during which time she might easily become pregnant. When she had her period a week after the honeymoon was over, we simply laughed it off and decided to try again.

Both of us are highly passionate people and we both need a lot of sexual intercourse. During those first few months it was like a long sexual spree, without end, because we were both desperately in love, physically turned on by one another and wanting to create a child. After three months, without anything happening, we went to a doctor. He suggested that we try a little longer. We tried for a couple of months more, then went back. The next step was to check us out. As usual, he started with me, giving me a bottle and saying to withdraw before orgasm and put my sperm into the jar.

Ann was beautiful that night. Instead of making me worry about withdrawal, she used her lips and then her hands during the climactic moments and managed to capture my sperm in the jar. A few days later we learned I couldn't have children.

This is quite a blow to a man; especially since I had always considered myself pretty much of a man. Add to that a very desperate need to have children of my own, and you can guess how it hit me. I took to drinking and one night, while in a rage, I happened to say that it wasn't right that she should be denied a child because I couldn't have one. I offered her a divorce. Of course she didn't take up the offer, but she did go to the doctor and demand he check her out.

We were lucky in one way, I guess; neither of us can have children. But for different reasons. I don't quite understand the medical reasons, though in simple terms she could become pregnant but would never be able to carry a child to birth.

Maybe it was a blessing, because neither of us is stopping some other person from having a child. I think that if you can't have children it is more just that you end up marrying somebody in the same situation. It was an accident with us; but a good one.

We thought about adoption, but I just didn't have the heart for it.

Our sex life became a little jagged for a while and I started drinking pretty heavily. I don't know why we didn't make love during this time, but we seemed to avoid such involvement for quite a long while. Oh, we made love a few times, like once a week, but more or less because both of us felt it was the right thing to do, not because we had any wild desire for sex after the shock of discovering we couldn't have babies. Strangely, it seemed pointless at that time.

I began to think that Ann didn't desire me any more, that maybe her sole reason for liking sex had been for the purpose of having children. I didn't have the heart to force sexual situations with Ann, and unless she made some kind of advance or it just happened by a set of circumstances, we just didn't make love; and even then it was pretty cold. This can drive a man wild, especially when he's had such a shock. I began to think Ann just didn't like sex; or didn't desire me. I didn't have the guts to come out and talk about it. In fact, all the starch had been knocked out of me.

There was a dark-haired woman working at the office, a divorcee who had always kidded with the men about sex, in a respectable way. Things like, if somebody happened to have a men's magazine, she'd open it to the centerfold, look at the girl and say: "Maybe I should pose for something like that."

She had a very good figure, big breasts, and wide hips. Her mouth was very wide and full and she had a way of looking into a guy's eyes like she was making a sexual offer.

I heard from one of the other guys that she was on the

make for sex, and one night when I had to work late, and she offered to stay and help me, I went along with the gag. I couldn't get my eyes off her body. She was wearing a sweater with buttons in front and a flaring skirt. Her breasts bulged against the sweater as if trying to pop the buttons. When the work was finished about nine, I suggested a drink. I had a bottle in my desk drawer and offered her a shot.

She sat on the small couch in my office, looked up at me, her legs spread provocatively, lips pouting into a pretty little smile. "Drink with a man and you don't know what might follow."

I laughed, but couldn't help thinking I really wanted to screw this cunt. She really turned me on. It was the first time I'd ever thought of another woman since knowing Ann. The whole thing shocked me right to the core. But I kept thinking it wouldn't really make any difference. Then my sex life was pretty terrible, too, I rationalized.

I fixed the drinks, saying: "I really need it."

She laughed, said: "You make that sound like you need something more than a drink."

I turned, said: "I'm a married man, you know."

"I really don't care. Do you?" This statement was pretty startling and I guess my face reflected my surprise. "Well," she said, "you have been looking at me like you'd like to tear off my sweater, bra, and...well, I guess you know what I mean."

I asked if it was that obvious.

She nodded as she took the drink. "I couldn't help but notice how you look at my boobs. I think it's nice. I like men to notice them. I think they're pretty good. It makes me feel real sexy. You make a girl get real sexy by just looking at her."

I saw right then it was going to be a long night at the office.

"You make a man feel pretty sexy, too," I admitted,

gulping on the raw whiskey.

'That nice I like making men feel sexy Is that wrong?" Her eyebrows arched very innocently

"Not if you like following through," I admitted, deciding to get on with it. I just didn't care any more. "Mere flirtation always seemed nothing but tease with nothing to back it up. Never liked that."

"If I find a man exciting and he finds me the same, I don't see why we shouldn't do something about it. As far as you being married is concerned, that's your problem. If you want something, I think a person should take it." Her words were fairly direct and promising. "So? What do you think about that?"

I leaned close to her and looked down at her body as if I were stripping it bare. "You've been asking for it," I said, reaching out and putting a hand on her large breast, "and I don't see any reason not to give it to you."

She laughed, delightedly and swiftly placed a hand on my penis, which was hard as hell. "I see little baby wants some pussy. Let's screw, Ralph. I'm really hot for you. I can't stand it any longer. Fuck here, right now."

It's funny how some girls can come on so strong and others will run like hell if you even suggest something sexy—just fast enough to exhaust you, then they'll fall into your arms.

This woman didn't seem to care what I thought of her, as long as I was overwhelmed by her sexuality. I guess she realized she'd built quite a reputation at the office and wanted just that.

At this point she stood, started unbuttoning her sweater. The sight of her large breasts tightly restrained against the white bra was really something to look at.

She said: "Don't worry about wearing anything, honey, because I take the pill and like to feel a man's prick naked in me. Does that shock you?"

"I don't shock easily."

"That's nice," she told me, thrusting out her bra-covered breasts. "Don't you think they're nice?"

"Beautiful," I assured her.

Then she undid the bra and her breasts bloomed out, full, supple, and beautifully self-supporting.

I stood, reached for her, cupping one breast in my right hand, fondling the nipple, which was very large, with a well-defined areola spreading out over the generous flesh.

I kissed her lips and they parted for my tongue. After that first embrace, her hands were between us, unzipping my pants. I squeezed her breasts to let her know I liked what her hands were doing.

She said: "I bet you're a breast man. I hope so. I like to be kissed and sucked there. I like sex, very much. You'll see!"

We helped each other get undressed and then came together in a standing position. She worked my penis between her thighs as we kissed, then after a few moments, while her legs were pressing and squeezing my hard, she said : "Suck my tits, lover, suck them real hard."

We lay down on the floor and I started feasting on her breasts, moving from one to the other while she caressed my erected shaft with gentle, searching fingers. Suddenly she got real hot and pulled my hard toward her crotch.

"Fuck it, love!" 'she demanded, spitting out the word in a low grunt.

It was the first time I'd heard a woman ever use that word in this manner and it was fantastically exciting. I shoved deep inside her cunt, which was moist and fiery, softly voluptuous as it folded about my shaft. She lifted up to take in the full extent.

Her hand gripped my shoulders and I gripped her wide hips. We took each other like two savage animals, hammering faster and faster. The orgasm was fantastic.

I fell away, lying on my back, overcome. But she hadn't finished. Sitting on me, so that her fanny was pressing my penis, she said: "Do me again! I don't want to stop now!" Her fanny rubbed back and forth on me until I started feeling erotic sensations. When she became aware of my excitement, she lifted up, pulled my shaft up against her moist pussy and worked the palm of her hand up and down on the bottom of my penis. It was highly stimulating and the minute I was really hard, she lifted up again and this time settled down into place, gulping my shaft into her hot tight cunt.

From then on she lifted up and down, up and down, real hard, real fast. Her lower lip tucked between her teeth as her face blanched in passion and lust. Little grunting sounds uttered from her throat and her large breasts pounded up and down. I gripped them in my hands and started squeezing and she cried, "Squeeze me hard, harder!"

It really turned me on and I squeezed as hard as she demanded.

That night when I got home I was exhausted. I'd found her sexing very exciting and the next day talked her into another session, but this time it was in a motel. I couldn't get enough of her.

She liked to talk dirty as hell, I soon learned. She'd say something like: "Suck my cunt, honey!" or "Bang my ass with your screwing cocky prick!" We carried on an affair for some weeks and the longer it continued the bolder she became. She would come into the office, when nobody else was around and grab my hand, shove it up her skirt and say: "My sexy cunt is burning." Or she might pass me in the hall and whisper in my ear: "Love, I need a big fat prick." Once when passing her in the hall she grabbed my arm, whispered: "Please, take me some place fast. I need it!"

Then she led me into a conference room. We locked the doors and she lifted up her skirt, pulled off her panties and leaned against the huge table, saying: "Feed that big fat screwing prick into me."

I unzipped myself and she gripped my shaft, worked it back and forth until it was real hard, and then pulled it towards her pussy. I entered and we savagely banged away until we'd had a mutual orgasm. Then quickly she put on her pants, smiled and said: "I'll be sorry when you stop giving it to me, you big ape!"

Like I said, it went on for several weeks, without stop.

I've gone into this much detail to show how impossible it would have been for any man to turn it off. As long as Ann didn't know, it couldn't hurt her. It wasn't cutting down on what she was getting, so what difference did it make? I just couldn't turn off.

I learned later that Ann guessed what was happening right from the first night and she went out the next day and picked up some man. We were both putting our marriage right on the rocks.

Then one night Ann came out and accused me of having an affair with one of the girls at the office. I couldn't lie. We argued for a short time; but there was something in her manner that bothered me. She didn't seem so hurt as worried. Then she admitted to having picked up some men. We had a real fight after that. If we hadn't really loved each other so much it might have ruined our marriage. The fact is that this forced us to consider our feelings for one another and our feelings about our marriage. We actually ended up making love, but not until a lot of soul searching. It was then that we realized that neither of us wanted a divorce. We accepted the fact that the shock of discovering we couldn't have children had been almost too much to take.

The result of it all was that we developed a pretty good sense of honesty about sex. From then on our bedroom sessions had returned to normal, taking in all the things we had done before marriage and also normal intercourse in Ann's vagina.

But some of the spark had gone. It was orgasm, love for sexual orgasm and giving to one another, but both of us suddenly realized that it wouldn't really hurt either of us if we enjoyed other partners. We talked about sex in a very open fashion.

I had learned there were such things as swapping partners and we decided to try this, in order to have a richer sex life. We had come to the conclusion that since we couldn't have babies, sex must be considered a thing of pleasure. We only lived once; we might as well make the most of our sexual impulses. Ann admitted to finding sexual intercourse with other men very exciting, though told me that to her I was the best. "It's only different, that's all."

It was necessary to talk to the girl I'd been having the affair with. I told her that Ann knew all about what had happened. She was pretty amazed at that. I said we were pretty well adjusted now, and that we had both decided that sex was a wonderful thing. We wanted to enjoy it in all its forms; we actually agreed there wasn't anything wrong with either of us having other partners. We both thought it might be fun if she and some other man came over for the night for a sex party. She really flipped. "You have quite a wife," she told me. I didn't bother to explain our real reasons. Neither of us wanted to adopt another person's child; we had decided to live a sensual, honest life and forget about children.

That first night, when we were all together, was trying for both Ann and myself. It had been a mistake having the girl I'd been screwing on the side as the second woman; yet there was a certain voluptuous pleasure in it all, too.

Ann didn't like her, and made it pretty obvious from the very beginning. But after a few stiff cocktails and conversation of a sexual nature, it was decided to get undressed, turn the lights off and use candles. The flames created flickering shadows and lovely highlights on the women's bodies. The two of them were obviously out to prove who was the best.

Ann made it a point to immediately start on the other man. She stepped up to him, reached below his balls and started fondling, saying: "My, you certainly have large balls. Is your prick as promising? Does it get real large and long and hard?"

I watched, fascinated, a little taken aback. Ann was pretty bold and blunt. It was the first time I'd seen her act this manner. In a way it was exciting, yet I felt a very great sense of awkwardness, even embarrassment. But the young girl from the office pressed her back against my fanny cheeks coming in contact with my penis. She gripped my hands against her breasts, then moved one hand down to her crotch, pressing it firmly in place. "Finger me, love," she suggested, working my index finger against the entrance to her vagina. "Like that. Sex me." And her fanny wiggled against my penis, which was beginning to respond.

I kept watching Ann. She was now holding the man's hard prick in her hands, rubbing it back and forth. He was toying with her pert, erect nipples. The sight of this scene was highly stimulating.

My girl said: "Ann, why don't you go down on it."

Ann ignored the remark. Instead she gripped the man's cock at its base and started moving the shaft up and down, so that the point was running along her sexual lips.

I felt my own shaft stiffening to a painful point of hardness and slipped it between the girl's thighs. She squeezed them together and rolled her hips. That sent wild erotic sensations through my whole body.

I saw Ann press her partner's prick to the entrance of her vagina and lift upwards on her tip-toes until his shaft penetrated to its base. A twitching convulsion of erotic fire ripped through me.

My girl now bent over, placing the palms of her I

hands on the floor and said: 'Stick me deep," in such a hot, erotic voice that I almost came from its sound mixed with the sight of my wife's face reacting in pleasure to what was so deeply thrust into her cunt.

Like a savage, all the time watching Ann, I shoved my shaft deep into the girl's moist sex hole and started hammering brutally at her as hard and fast as I could; almost beating her with my penis. I think I was torn between orgiastic excitement and a little bit of jealousy. That is common the first time you do what we were doing.

Yet the orgiastic pleasure of my climax was overwhelming. I just kept watching the expression on Ann's face as she responded to the little thrusting jerks the man was making with his hips. She was still standing in front of him, breasts hugged against his chest, arms about his neck, legs wrapped about his legs. The full weight of her body seemed to be on his prick. He was actually doing no more than bouncing up and down in little jerking movements, just enough to make some friction between their sexual organs.

To this day I think I climaxed for Ann and at the same time.

We did other things that night, but we've done those and more since, with other couples. We have swapped with many couples.

I met Jimmy and became quick friends. We talked about sex and when he learned that Ann and I liked to switch partners we arranged a thing to work Laura around to the idea. For some time we'd get together on week-ends and have sex parties. Sometimes at the apartments, several times going to the mountains or the beach, staying in connected rooms or in a cabin, and having wild orgies.

It was during this time that I learned the pleasure of having more than one woman make over my body. I find it highly exciting to be lapping it up—going down on one woman while another is riding my penis.

I remember one night at the house when Nancy was going down on me, Jimmy hitting her pussy with his hard shaft and Laura standing so that I could hold her hips and make love to her with my lips and tongue. It was really something and I was turned on like wild. By the time Nancy had given me a real good working over, I just kept going at Laura and this excited me into another erection.

I moved the two of us back and then sat Laura on the end of a table and coupled with her. She went simply mad, crazy-mad with passion as I penetrated her pussy. She cried out real loud, gripping me with her fingers, clutching to my shoulders like a cat. I knew she'd had a couple of climaxes while I was performing cunnilingus, but she climaxed almost immediately upon my entrance. That convulsive gripping about my shaft sent a quick come through it, but we didn't stop, just continued shoving our hips together. We climaxed a short time again, almost at the same time and Laura was spent out.

Nancy came over to me and went down on her knees, took hold of my now pretty limp shaft and said: "You have any more of it left for little old me?" And the way her fingers pulled along my shaft sent a tingle through my whole body. She murmured in delight and started feeding on my penis until it gained a full erection. Then she lay back on the floor, opened her legs and looking up at me, said: "Screw it good, Ralph!"

As I entered her, Dave said he wanted part of the action and straddled her face and she went ape, hips grinding wildly on my shaft while her lips went to work on his. I lasted a long time and that session burned in my memory for days afterwards. That's the kind of things we can do!

That's the basics about living together, three couples, all sexually driven to explore any position and any type of sexual thrill that a man and woman can experience; it's sex-time any time you want it, in any fashion.

I don't say that it gets boring doing it the conventional

way with *one* woman, but I will say this: You get to the point where it's just not enough.

There have been times when I can't get enough of female pussy and one woman isn't enough at one time.

We've played some pretty wild games. I made a bet, once, that I could give all three girls a climax without running out of power.

So the girls stripped naked, lay on the floor, side by side, but when I joined them, they really turned on me, like a unit, all team-working together to knock me out. It was really something. The others watched.

I had my hands on Ann's and Laura's crotch, caressing and fingering, while Nancy lowered her head between my legs. The other two girls started running their hands all over me, caressing my body in such a way that it was almost as stimulating as what Nancy was doing with her lips.

When I was high up, like a pole, the girls lowered me on my back and Nancy lowered herself onto my shaft. It was really something trying to keep from having an orgasm right off. But I relaxed and just took in the sensation of her moist embrace pulling up and down on my hotstick, then suddenly she climaxed, lifted away and Laura took her place. Laura is smaller and her pussy is tighter and I just went off like a fountain deep inside her the minute my shaft had penetrated to its full extent. She laughed and then started to really screw her hips around and around, up and down, faster and faster as my shaft hardened in her tight grasp. When she climaxed I almost went with her, but fought it off. Then when Ann replaced her, I relaxed in the sweet awareness that this was my wife, the woman I had married; and we really made a session out of it. I think both of us were exhausted by the time we both climaxed at the same time. I felt myself losing control, then Ann suddenly moaned, shoved down against me real hard and shuddered convulsively with her whole body as I exploded like an atomic bomb, deep within her.

Now tell me, how can a guy get such a beautiful experience with only one woman? The fantastic thing about this was the fact that everything led up to Ann and the total expression and experience of emotional love. Nancy and Laura had served to merely warm me up for Ann.

Like I said, even before I got married I liked women and what their bodies could give. Finding Ann and getting married had been more than mere love of a woman and more than merely the desire to have children. But to be quite honest, the shock of discovering we couldn't have children jarred us up quite a bit. And it changed our attitudes about life and what our function in life should be, I guess.

To be quite honest, I'm not one to live on deep thoughts. I've found it is easier to just *live,* get out of life as much as you can. Living with two other couples has changed our habit patterns, but I believe for the best. We can have just about any kind of sexual experience we decide is desirable. If you aren't going to have children around—and we thought of adoption but rejected that idea because neither of us wanted some other person's child—then there just doesn't seem any reason not to live with our guts. We aren't hurting anybody in the way we live.

When I think back on my life and look forward into the future, I realize that we've made the best decision. We have a kind of family union but with spades. I'm married, but not only to Ann, but to Laura and Nancy, to a lesser degree. It's better than swapping partners, which we did for some time, getting together with other married couples. But that seemed pretty shallow compared to what we have here. When you swap wives with another guy, it's cold-blooded. You get together and then the other wife clutches to you. Then you go into one of the bedrooms, get undressed and start sexing it. One wife wanted to examine my sexual parts in detail, saying it was interesting to see the difference between her husband and other men. But, while this kind of examination was quite sexual and stimulating, since she used first her fingers, then her lips and tongue, it was a little cold. We had orgasm together. That was all.

The way we are living now with the other two couples, it's something far more intimate. We all know each other and there are times when either Nancy or Laura actually request that we go to bed and sex it up because they desire me; *knowing what it is like!*

In a way it is like being married to three women and there is at least one woman who will want sex at any one time; willing to give you a sexual ball upon request. There aren't any of these moody times, once a month times that a husband gets all hung-up with when his wife has her period. Hell, there are two other girls to pick from. And to say nothing about an orgy where more than two of us are involved in some kind of sexual play together. It is always experimental, always attempting to find a new way, or new combinations of ways, to make the sex scene more exciting.

For me, and I guess for everybody else at the house, it's the only way to make life logical in this modern world. It's better than pure simple marriage and it's better than wife-swapping. What else can I say about it? Except that other people should try it; they'd be surprised what rewards it can give to their life.

COMMENTS

I think of the three couples; Ralph and Ann's marriage and experience is probably the most tragic, for they tried for a normal married life and almost made it, only to be toppled by the inability to have children. The bitterness of this shock was revealed by how they reacted so violently to it. Why they didn't adopt children is really difficult to

say; most people adjust to such disappointment and continue to live normal married lives. I think that Ralph is a
classic example of a man who is not sure of his manhood
and once he discovered it was impossible to have children
he took this as another attack at his perverted fears about
himself. To look at Ralph one could hardly think of him as
doubting his manhood, yet his actions and the reactions of
others to him, seem to indicate this as a very strong possibility.

I talked briefly to Ann, who didn't wish to say much
about her personal life. She *did* reveal this much: "Why
lie? We tried the straight marriage bit. We found it was
impossible to have children. It shattered our whole concept
of marriage and made the old ideas of morality seem foolish and meaningless. I discovered I didn't care any more
about anything. *That was my first reaction.* Then we
started toying with the swapping thing and it seemed right.
I did have a few one night stands with pick-ups. That was
how far down I'd gone.

"Our marriage was almost finished. This life we live
now has saved the marriage and I guess we could say it
has saved our lives in more ways than one. Surely Ralph
told you all there is to say. I really don't wish to talk about
it. I'd rather live one day at a time and just enjoy what is
probably my way of escaping ugly hard truths about life
and myself. Is that clear enough?"

Her bitterness reflected an attempt to escape, *in toto*! I
think this was Ralph's partial motive. For some people it is
easier to escape reality than to face it and the world, as
mature adults. Both Ralph and Ann struck this reporter as
being this kind of people.

To a certain degree the others were escape-prone, as
David pointed out in a short conversation with me, the
only one in private he would give.

"I grew up thinking sex was part of romance. With
Nancy it was just that. I'd had a few women before her. I

respected Nancy right from the beginning because I could see something in her eyes that seemed haunted and...well, desperate for love. The affair that followed in time was a logical thing; our living together either developed into marriage or something else. Then something else has turned out to be this. It isn't the best of all possible worlds, but it is, to me, and I guess to the others, a way of rebelling against a world that seems all wrong. If you are living in a kind of hell that might destroy itself at any moment, either in a personal way or in a mass explosion, you either ignore the possibility or you decide to make the most of what you got. I don't want to get married to any woman right now, because I've found something better than singular union with only one woman. There is a certain amount of freedom in our sexual orgy games. We don't have to think, we don't have to worry—it is complete escape. And for me, at least, this is a desirable state of affairs.

"Maybe it is escaping from reality—not maturing as some psychologists might claim—but everybody has their own means of ignoring their own, or the world's, hell. Some drink themselves to death; some don't relate to any other human being, or simply screw every pick-up they can get; some turn away from love and sex and live hellish lives; some go homosexual just for kicks; some kill or rob; some take dope. You name it and it's done.

"We seek escape from the hard part of the world by inter-relating between ourselves, six human beings who find sexual and emotional union between each other as a fulfilling reward for facing the day to day world of reality. As they say, everybody has a right to pick their own poison. *We've picked our own form, or our means, of survival.* And as long as we aren't hurting anyone, what's the beef?"

While their way of living and "facing reality"—escaping—is not mine, I did find that Dave's statement was probably the best defense for their moral attitudes and sexual actions. The question which seemed most important to all was in effect: Why should they be damned for what they do when the world at large is guilty of far greater crimes over which it doesn't even bat an eye? Murder and war and violence and hate are far greater sins than having a sexual orgy every night of the year; is the reasoning!

If it might not be our answer, our idea of morality, we must ask ourselves, first, is ours any better? Is it better to be married to one person and cheat, going behind their backs to another lover: or better to live openly with other couples, sharing each other in a total manner, in home, body and emotions?

Probably like all judgments and all morality held by each person, none of it is completely moral or completely true and just. Probably there is no black or white judgment but only the acceptance of oneself as a total human being, made up of grays, or a mixture of all colors, admitting one's weaknesses as well as strengths and trying to make the best out of this life.

These people I talked to, in order to put this book together, were trying their own personal experiment in order to find the answer to happiness.

It isn't my answer, and possibly not the reader's. But it is the answer to them and many like them, some who live like the Hippies and Beats. Morality must be questioned only by those of us who are perfect—sinless.

I personally know nobody who is perfect enough. who is spotless of all sin; or morally clean enough to make a final and just decision of what is right and what is wrong. Each person must judge for themselves, but with the admission that no judgment, no code of ethics, no morality is perfect.

In closing I would like to point out the following facts that I observed in talking to and knowing these people.

None, at any time, gave any suggestion that they felt it was their moral and God-like duty to tell others what they should or shouldn't do.

None of the women made even the slightest pass at me or indicated that they would even consider doing so with me or anybody other than those people who believe in the same things they do.

David made one observation on this matter. "We have it made, according to our own personal beliefs. We find it totally unnecessary to seek other partners, outside of our private little fold of social contacts. There is no need for it, simply because we have found a good answer. We are free; and in the freedom comes the reality and realization that once you are free you are content; happy! Or at least as happy as possible. As for the few parties we give, with other friends who believe as we do, well, that's just a normal by-product of our lives. And probably because of that we don't have any hang-ups about sex."

They have what many couples who are married have: they are loyal to their own loves and beliefs, they give as much as they take, they help each other in times of need.

Is this what will come, as Jimmy suggested, in the future world when we are over-populated and have to share living quarters with other couples? It is my personal hope that other solutions will be found by that time, yet I can't help but wonder.

Do their lives give us a peek into the future lives of our children or their children? If so, maybe then there will be couples who are strangely mal-adjusted to *their* society and will try to build a life for themselves, a private, anti-social life, where they will want to share themselves only with each other, until death. Will they seem as perverse to their fellow men as these six people might seem to us? Or will there come a time when man can live the kind of life he wants, no matter what it might involve, just as long as nobody is hurting?

Will there ever come a time when each person can find his or her own code of ethics, own personal morality, and live the kind of life which will give them the greatest pos-sible happiness, without others pointing a figure and creat-ing names like perverse, degenerate, immoral?

As Shakespeare wrote four hundred years ago:

Men at some times are masters of their fates: The fault, dear Brutus, is not in our stars, But in ourselves, that we are underlings!

PLURAL SEX, BY CARSON DAVIS

ABOUT THE AUTHOR

Carson Davis is just another pen name for a rather prolific writer who had many other pen names and scores of books published during his writing career.

The author reports that he started out as a writer of fiction, and that the really hungry market, which existed when he began writing, was the so-called "adult novels" aimed at male sexual fantasies. Much like the later, and sometimes even racier, historical and romantic pocketbooks for females, which became the rage of the publishing field for decades, they were on the racy side. Today they would be rather mild Mature-Rated stories, R at worse. Though there were those members of society that considered them X-rated from page one all the way through to the very last period.

When he began writing such books some of the publishers would get into nasty legal battles with the local District Attorneys out to pacify voters during elections. Such censorship cases never amounted to much; and the laws of the land supported the publishers.

When the Carson Davis books first appeared in print, they were rather X-rated in many ways, but today would probably deserve a strong R rating. In fact a six-volume hardcover edition of the "best of Carson Davis" appeared in Europe, in both Dutch and French translations, with some minor censorship insofar as some terms used in these

145

original editions. Those books were certainly just R rated even by their standards back then.

Today Wildside Press is offering a few of Mr. Davis' books to its readership. The realistic grounding of his work is starkly evident. And his continual message reflects a non-judgmental attitude about people's moral ethics.

He writes:

"I have lived in Southern California most of my life, and perhaps that has molded my own personal convictions concerning morality. I've experienced marriage in a wonderful way. And much like my Carson Davis, have been convinced that real love and commitment comes when people are willing to share their lives together in an honest and loving manner. How that shapes itself is a matter of each person's belief and standards. And as long as they are consenting adults not hurting anybody by their actions, that's all the truly matters in the end.

"These books under the Carson Davis byline have always been an especially rewarding experiment, for they gave me a chance to express a lot of basic thoughts and ideas which can't be expressed in novels in exactly the same way. In these books I was able to examine ideas and concepts that reached wide across many cultural and religious borders. The only restriction was the theme of each book. Within that boundary there were no limits, and I had some professional advice that made it possible to keep a very seriously sound underlining hard truth behind each and every case history story related. I always felt that all of these books contained a very real hard truth about life, sex, relationships and some important insights into a wide array of human thinking concerning our lives.

"I have never talked to a person who was a real pervert or deviant, but rather to many people with different points of view who had something to reveal in their apparent "confessions" about life, sex and what they believed

was the ideal solution to just surviving.

"It is enough to say these books were popular and have found circulation throughout the world. They stand up today as well as they did when originally published."

.

www.ingramcontent.com/pod-product-compliance
Lightning Source LLC
Chambersburg PA
CBHW020004290326
41935CB00007B/302